The
come
as you are
Workbook

A Practical Guide to the Science of Sex

Emily Nagoski, Ph.D.

Simon & Schuster Paperbacks

New York London Toronto Sydney New Delhi

Simon & Schuster Paperbacks
An Imprint of Simon & Schuster, LLC.
1230 Avenue of the Americas
New York, NY 10020

First Simon & Schuster trade paperback edition June 2019

SIMON & SCHUSTER PAPERBACKS and colophon are
registered trademarks of Simon & Schuster, LLC.

For information about special discounts for bulk purchases,
please contact Simon & Schuster Special Sales
at 1-866-506-1949 or business@simonandschuster.com.

The Simon & Schuster Speakers Bureau can bring authors to your live event.
For more information or to book an event, contact the
Simon & Schuster Speakers Bureau at 1-866-248-3049 or
visit our website at www.simonspeakers.com.

Interior design by Ruth Lee-Mui

Manufactured in the United States of America

12   13   14   15   16   17   18   19   20

Library of Congress Cataloging-in-Publication Data has been applied for.

ISBN 978-1-9821-0732-1

contents

Introduction   vii

part one: the (not-so-basic) basics

1. Anatomy: No Two Alike   3
2. The Dual Control Model   20
3. Context   39

part two: sex in context

4. Emotional Context   73
5. Cultural Context   94

part three: sex in action

6. Arousal   119
7. Desire   136

part four: ecstasy for everybody

8. **Orgasm**   161
9. **A New Script**   181

Conclusion   199
Acknowledgments   201
Recommended Reading   203

introduction

This workbook has one job: to provide practical, evidence-based tools to enhance your personal sexual wellbeing. If you want to develop a better relationship with your own sexuality, reduce your frustration or worry about sex, or maximize your access to sexual pleasure, you're in the right place. If you want to understand who you are as a sexual person, why your sexual arousal, desire, and pleasure are what they are, and how you can begin removing the obstacles that stand between you and great sex, you, too, are in the right place! Welcome! In these pages you'll find exercises, information, and tools that can deepen your understanding of your own sexual wellbeing and help you communicate clearly with your partner(s) about sex in ways that empower you to explore.

In the last few decades, the science of women's sexuality has clarified our understanding of how sex works. When seen through a scientist's careful eye rather than through a distorting cultural lens, every aspect of women's sexuality—from arousal to desire to orgasm—defies all preconceptions. While this workbook is written for women (i.e., people who identify as women) and is based on the science of women's sexuality, people of any gender can use almost every tool and activity in it. That's by design, because everyone, of every gender, deserves to have great sex. Also, great sex comes from appreciating your sexuality *and* your partner's sexuality, and sometimes your partner isn't a woman.

There are some things this workbook doesn't offer. If you are looking for in-depth explanations of the science of sexuality, read my first book, *Come As You Are* (*CAYA*). If you want to learn "techniques" for giving great oral sex or otherwise enhancing your sexual performance, you'll find those at www.goodinbed.com. And if you're hoping for an academic exploration of the cultural or political structures that constrain and police women's sexuality, there are lots of books that offer that, but this is not one of them. This workbook's one job is to help you enhance your relationship with your own sexuality.

how the workbook is organized

The workbook is organized similarly to *CAYA*. If you've read *CAYA*, you'll find this workbook deepens your understanding of the science of sexuality as it applies to your personal sex life. But even if you haven't read *CAYA*, the workbook can help you maximize your sexual wellbeing and facilitate better communication about sex.

It is divided into four parts. Part 1, "The (Not-So-Basic) Basics," is about the fundamental hardware of sexuality: your body, your brain, and your context. Part 2, "Sex in Context," delves deeply into the aspects of your life that influence your sexuality: stress and culture. Part 3, "Sex in Action," offers the science of sexual arousal and desire as an alternative to the cultural messages you explored in Part 2. And finally, Part 4, "Ecstasy for Everybody," moves beyond the science of arousal and desire to the science of pleasure and satisfaction.

Throughout the book, you'll find questions from my "Q & A Vault." At many events, organizers provide a box—it might be an empty, decorated tissue box or, one time, an actual miniature mailbox—into which people can drop anonymous questions. Over the years, I've accumulated a lot of these, written on scraps of paper, hotel stationery, paper napkins, and note cards. At the close of the event, I pull out the questions and answer them all, one by one. This workbook includes verbatim questions I've been asked by real people just like you, with the answers I gave the audience.

You can use the workbook on your own or with a partner; independently or with the support of a coach or therapist. Use it however feels right for you. Each chapter concludes with a "One Important Thing" exercise, to help you clarify your thinking and experience.

effective brainstorming

Several exercises in the workbook call for "brainstorming," which means generating a lot of ideas and writing them down, without judging whether they're good or bad. Some people are naturally good at it and enjoy doing it.

If you're not one of those people, here's an analogy that might help. Brainstorming is like the tryouts for junior high cheerleading. At those tryouts, there are two unbreakable rules:

1.   Everyone—that is, every idea—is allowed to audition. Of course not everyone will make the squad, but only if you allow everyone, absolutely everyone, to audition do you

discover the hidden gem, the shy new girl who, though you'd never know it to look at her, can do splits and backflips and yells like a banshee. Before you see her, you have to let every single kid, from the popular girls to the goth and emo kids to the math team, have their turn.

2. Tryouts have a time limit. You set a timer and you let the chaos happen, then when the timer goes off, you're done. Don't keep brainstorming until you find the "right" answer. Sometime you can't know which answer is right until you spend more time with the promising ones.

So to brainstorm effectively, set a time limit (just a few minutes!), and then write down literally everything that comes to mind, whether it seems right or not—whether it even seems relevant or not. It's normal to think of something and then automatically evaluate it, asking yourself, "But is that true? Is that what I mean?" or "Doesn't this idea contradict that other idea I just wrote down?" Set those evaluative thoughts to one side for the moment. You'll go through the editorial process later. Assume that somewhere between 50 and 90 percent of the ideas you generate when brainstorming will never lead to anything. Those ideas are not a waste! Their role in the brainstorm is to *get out of the way*, to step back and become a crowd that oohs and aahs when the hidden gems appear. And they can only serve that purpose if you include them. Write them down.

a note about relationships

This workbook's focus is on helping you, the individual reader, understand and maximize your own personal sexual wellbeing. This includes developing skills for communicating with a partner about sex, but relationship skills more generally are mostly outside the scope of this workbook. Many great resources focus on relationship skills. Strongly evidence-based approaches for creating stable, happy relationships include John Gottman's *The Seven Principles for Making Marriage Work* and Sue Johnson's *Hold Me Tight.* But the starting point in this workbook—and, I think, in many women's experience of great sex—is developing a stable, happy relationship with your own personal sexuality.

If there's one lesson I've learned during my decades working as a sex educator, it's that a woman's best source of wisdom and insight into her sexual wellbeing is *her own internal experience.* Sometimes our partners can be valuable mirrors, helping us to notice our internal experience. But sometimes we must sit quietly with our own bodies, hearts, and minds, and allow our inner voice to speak its truth directly to us. My hope is that this workbook will help you do just that.

Are you ready?

Deep breath. Soften your shoulders. Relax your jaw. Let yourself smile a little.

And let's get started.

part one

the (not-so-basic) basics

one

anatomy: no two alike

On the day you were born—or maybe even sooner—the adults around you looked at the body parts between your legs and declared, "It's a girl!" or "It's a boy!"

In that moment, your gender was assigned and your caregivers began to calibrate and organize their expectations for what toys you'd play with, what moods you'd have, whom you'd love, and how you'd love them. That assigned gender even shaped their expectations about how you should feel about the very body parts on which they based those expectations. And if they said, "It's a girl," chances are those expectations include some pretty toxic crap.

I'll illustrate with two very different stories.

First, a woman told me about watching her grown-up brother changing his baby daughter's diaper. When she was clean and ready for her fresh diaper, the little girl reached down and touched her genitals, and Dad said, "Ah-ah! Don't touch that!"

How would he have reacted if his baby had touched her belly button?

How would he have reacted if his baby had a penis instead?

What lesson is that little girl learning about how she's supposed to feel about her body? And how do you feel about the idea of her learning it?

It's one tiny moment in her life, one that she will not remember. But it accumulates with uncountable other tiny moments, teaching her that her body isn't really hers to do with as she pleases, it's a foreign object to be avoided, a source of shame.

The second story provides a contrast. A therapist at one of my trainings told me a story about her two-year-old daughter. The therapist said, "She was on her bouncy ball and she started rocking and rubbing herself on the ball, and she said, 'Mommy, this feels good!' and I said, 'Yes, honey, that's your clitoris,' and she said, 'My clitoris is my *favorite*!'"

What did that little girl learn about how she's supposed to feel about her body?

What do you notice yourself feeling about the idea of her learning that lesson?

Few of us grew up with such clear messages about bodily autonomy. Most of us were raised, intentionally or not, with messages of *shame*. The shame is rooted deeply in our culture. Even the medical term for the "It's a girl" package of genitals— "pudendum"—is derived from the Latin *pudere*, meaning "to make ashamed," named for "the shamefacedness that is in women to have them seen."

But our culture is not our ultimate source of knowledge about our sexuality. Our own body is. When we can tune into its messages without judgment or fear; when we can see it on its own terms; when we can listen to its signals about wants and likes, what it dreads and dislikes—we can communicate more clearly with partners, access greater pleasure, and transform how we live in the world as sexual people.

In this chapter, you'll try some evidence-based strategies that challenge and release the negative feelings about your genitals that so many of us absorb early in our lives. Many of them are exercises that were part of my training as a sex educator. Others are assignments sex therapists sometimes "prescribe" to their clients. All of them are optional. And all of them begin to shift the very foundation on which your relationship with your sexuality is built, because our relationship with our sexual bodies is the foundation of our relationship with sex itself.

No Two Alike for Transgender, Intersex, and Nonbinary Folks

For cisgender people—that is, those whose personal experience of their gender matches the gender they were assigned at birth ("It's a girl!")— I generally recommend befriending their genitals, treating them with the same kindness and playful affection they have for their best friend. But if you're someone whose personal experience of gender doesn't match the gender you were assigned—if you're transgender, intersex, or nonbinary—you may feel great about your "factory direct" parts, or you might have a different kind of relationship with your genitals and other gendered body characteristics.* It's not uncommon for trans, intersex, and nonbinary people to experience some feelings of resentment

*S. Bear Bergman starts all of his Sex Positive Trans Sex workshops with a helpful and validating reminder to attendees that I have always appreciated. He says, "Just to be very, very clear: no matter how you feel about your genitals or any other body parts, it doesn't make you more or less transgender/nonbinary/genderqueer. Your gender identity and your feelings about your genitals are both 100 percent valid."

or even grief about their gendered body parts. And if those parts have also been subject to traumatic experiences in medical (and other) contexts, they may be associated with big, uncomfortable emotions. Those are completely valid feelings, and they can result in a relationship with your genitals that, even on a good day, may be more similar to your feelings about an unpleasant work colleague you just need to tolerate.

Feel free to skip this chapter altogether if you prefer not to go there right now. Or you can replace or supplement the exercises in this chapter with the following two practices that some folks find helpful, and continue through the workbook from there. I hope these exercises make the start of this book feel less alienating for you.

1. **Give your parts names that feel right for you.** One trans woman I know calls her genitals her strapless, and if asked why, says "She's not a strap-on, she's a strapless," complete with a runway-worthy flourish. When I saw sex educator S. Bear Bergman brainstorm with a group of students about words they liked for their own erogenous zones, one trans man said he called his genitals "Buck Rogers." Why? It felt right to him.

   Finding words that feel right for you isn't just about building a healthy (if still difficult) relationship with your body. Vocabulary that feels safe and/or sexy can help you communicate with your partner(s) about how and where you like to be touched and even help you access less stressful (or less traumatizing) medical care. A competent and aware medical provider can use your preferred terms instead of the heavily gendered medicalized words, if you can tell them which words feel safer for you.

2. **Begin a practice of lovingkindness toward your body.** You may feel fine about your body and its many parts, or you might feel frustrated or upset about it (or both, or other things instead, or all of those things at once sometimes). It's very common that trans, nonbinary, and intersex people have complicated relationships with their bodies. A practice of lovingkindness isn't about "learning to love your body" so much as it is a way of wishing it well. Feel welcome and encouraged to wish peace and ease to body parts that you hope someday to say farewell to (So long! Pleasant journey!) and that you hope someday to welcome (Travel safely to me!), as well as the ones you currently have.

"Hello, [name]. May you know kindness. May you know love. May you know peace. May you be at ease."

say the words

A lot of us can't even say the word for a specific genital part without feeling awkward—just seeing the words on these pages might "squick" some readers. Squick is an emotional reaction of withdrawal, avoidance, or disgust. If even letters on a page make us want to turn away, how in the world can we turn toward the parts themselves with kindness and compassion? In this activity, you'll practice living with the anatomical names for genital parts.

Sometimes the easiest way to begin practicing this activity is to try saying nongenital body parts. Try it with these three words—just read them slowly and notice, with curiosity and without judging, any thoughts, emotions, or physical sensations they bring up:

Elbow

Tongue

Skin

Pause and take a moment to write down any thoughts, emotions, or physical sensations they bring up:

Now try it with these four words—just read them slowly to yourself and notice any thoughts, emotions, or physical sensations they bring up as you read them silently:

Vagina
Vulva
Labia
Clitoris

Pause again and take a moment to write down any thoughts, emotions, or physical sensations they bring up:

Next, I invite you to say the words out loud as you read them, saying each word very, very softly, even whispering it, like you're whispering a secret "I love you" to your soul mate, and notice, with curiosity and without judgment, any thoughts, feelings, or physical sensations that brings up. Whispering "I love you" to your soul mate, say:

Vagina
Vulva
Labia
Clitoris

Pause for a moment and write down any thoughts, emotions, or physical sensations brought up by saying these words aloud:

Now try saying it conversationally, like someone just said hello to you, and you're saying hello in return. Again, just notice with curiosity and without judgment any thoughts, feelings, or physical sensations that brings up. Saying hello, say:

Vagina
Vulva
Labia
Clitoris

Pause and take a moment to write down any thoughts, emotions, or physical sensations they bring up:

And finally, try saying it like you're saying, "Hooray!" because you just heard the best news in the world!

Vagina!
Vulva!
Labia!
Clitoris!

Pause and take a moment to write down any thoughts, emotions, or physical sensations they bring up:

all the same parts, organized in different ways

Every set of genitals is made of the same basic parts as everyone else's, but they're organized in a unique way, so the appearance of everyone's genitals is completely unique—beautiful and glorious and just as lovely as every other set of genitals.

Your task in this exercise is to find and look at diverse images of genitals. Yes, it is possible to find positive and diverse images of genitals on the Internet! Look at the genitals you see there with curiosity and nonjudgment.

Here are a few phrases to search for, to get you started:

- Fucking Like a Feminist
- Our Danish Sisters
- *I'll Show You Mine*, by Wrenna Robertson
- Visual Vaginal Library

As you search for and look at diverse, positive images of genitals, notice what emotions you experience. Write down what the experience was like:

identify your parts

This exercise is a treasure hunt of sorts. In a space where you feel safe and comfortable, take off your clothes, get a hand mirror, and look at your vulva.

"Vulva" is the anatomical name for the "it's a girl" package of external genitals. Most of us call the vulva the vagina, but technically the vagina is the internal reproductive canal. I believe that the names we call things says something about our priorities; calling it the vagina erases the clitoris completely and reduces our sexual anatomy to its reproductive function. When we call each part by its proper name, we open up space for a more complete picture of our sexuality. After all, you would never call your face your throat.

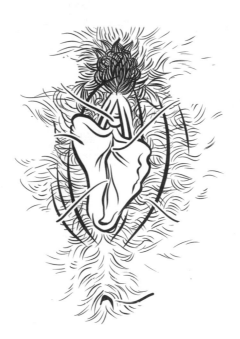

Look at your genitals in a mirror and see if you can identify these parts:

- *Labia majora ("big lips")*—The outer folds of the vulva, with stretchy skin, where hair grows.
- *Labia minora ("little lips")*—The internal folds of the vulva, which may be large or small, pink or brown, or a gradient blend of both. Not everyone with a vulva has these, and others have "little lips" that are actually larger than the "big" .outer lips.
- *Clitoris*—Technically it's called the "glans clitoris" (the head of the clitoris). It's the nub just below the cleft of your labia. It might be easier to find it manually than visually. Start with the tip of your middle finger at the cleft where your labia divide. Press down gently, wiggle your finger back and forth, and scoot your fingertip slowly down between your labia until you feel a flexible cord under the skin. It might help to pull your skin taut by tugging upward on your pubic bone with your free hand. It might also help to lubricate your finger with spit, commercial lube, some allergen-free hand cream, or even a little coconut oil.
- *Urethral opening*—Between the clitoris and the vagina, you'll find the opening of the urethra. It may be obvious, or it may be subtle, almost invisible.
- *Vaginal opening*—South of the urethral opening is the vagina. It is the opening itself that's sensitive to erotic sensations, not so much the internal canal.

You'll find an "answer sheet"—a vulva illustration with labels—at the end of the chapter.

What emotions do you experience looking at your genitals? What kind of relationship do you have with them? Friend? Foe? Family? Frenemy? Stranger you're meeting for the first time? Write down what the experience was like:

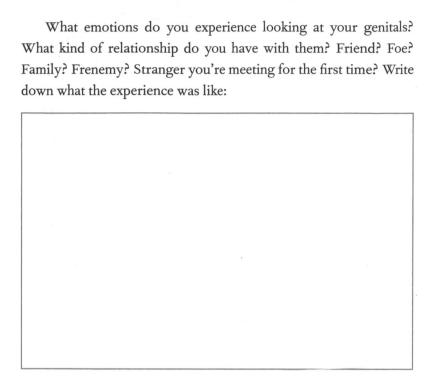

Bonus exercise: Do this activity again when you are very sexually aroused and notice how your genitals look then!

Meeting your genitals face-to-face might be difficult if you experience genital pain, which makes your genitals a source of suffering for you. Women in particular are taught that pain is just "expected" with sex. It is not. If you are experiencing unwanted genital pain, talk to a medical provider.

It's sadly true that many nonspecialist medical providers are taught the same thing as the rest of us, that pain is "normal" (again: it is not), so some providers may be unhelpful or even dismissive. How do you find a *great* provider if you're experiencing pelvic pain? When I asked some great providers where I can refer people, they named the Herman & Wallace Pelvic Rehabilitation Institute at www.pelvicrehab.com.

Just about everything we experience related to sexuality is normal—all the same parts, organized in different ways—except pain. Pain is your body asking for help. You deserve pain-free sex, and effective treatments are available.

from the q & a vault

Q: I am very conscious of the look of my labia. My inner labia are very long and hang below the outer. I always want to tuck them in. Always worried about what my partners think. What really is normal? Sometimes I think I should have them removed. Help!

A: As long as you're not experiencing pain, your parts are normal. Genitals come in a vast range of shapes, sizes, colors, and configurations, and they're all normal. They're all made of the same parts as everyone else's.

I know that somewhere or other you were told there's one specific way a vulva should look, and if it doesn't look that way, there's something wrong. In fact, just as women's bodies are Photoshopped to look impossibly "perfect" in magazines, women's genitals in porn magazines may be digitally altered to look more like a closed clamshell. But all genitals are made of the same parts, just organized in different ways, so there's no such thing as a vulva that needs surgery to make it "look normal." It is already normal. Actually, it's not just normal, it's beautiful, in all its uniqueness.

And if a partner has any response other than "Wow!" and "Hooray!" at the sight of your beautiful vulva, maybe you want to teach them how misguided they are . . . or maybe you just don't want to grant them the privilege of seeing your beautiful vulva.

I want to live in a world where everyone's body belongs to them, and they get to choose what they do with it and how they feel about it. I want every one of you to feel you have a choice about how to feel about your body and your sexuality.

Can it be done? Can a grown-up learn to turn toward her own body with confidence and joy? Oh yes. You can start creating that world now, simply by owning your own parts, owning the names of those parts, and beginning to shed the cultural meaning imposed on them, replacing that meaning with their true, biological meaning: everyone's made of the same parts, organized in different ways.

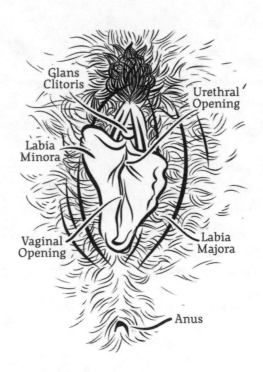

one important thing

Take a moment to look back at the exercises in this chapter. Write down one important thing you learned, whether it's about sex in general or about your sexuality in particular:

two

the dual control model

You might think sexual response happens between your legs, but it turns out where the action really happens is between your ears— and it's not as simple as most of us have been led to believe.

The mechanism in your brain that governs sexual response has *two* main parts. You can think of it like driving a car. One part is a sexual gas pedal or accelerator that notices all the sex-related stimuli—everything you see, hear, smell, touch, taste, think, feel, or believe—and sends the "turn-on" signal. It's functioning at a low level all the time. Even now, as you're reading this, a little bit of "turn-on" signal is being sent.

The other part is the sexual brakes, which notice all the good reasons not to be turned on right now—everything you see, hear, smell, touch, taste, think, feel, or believe that your brain interprets as a potential threat—and send the "turnoff" signal. The brakes, too, function at a low level all the time. Anything happening around you right now that makes it an inappropriate time to be aroused—the people you may be with, the location you're in, the stress you may be experiencing, even how you feel about your body and your sexuality—can keep the brakes on.

So the process of becoming aroused is the dual process of turning on all the ons and turning off all the offs. Which means:

1. It's 100 percent normal to experience *ambivalence* around sex. For example, you might like the way your partner is kissing your neck, but not like that it's happening in the middle of a party. Or you might not love the way they're kissing your neck but really enjoy that it's happening in public.

2. Sometimes one stimulus can both hit the brake and activate the accelerator at the same time, particularly if you've learned that sexuality is itself a threat. If you tried to drive a car with one foot on the accelerator and one foot on the brake, how would that go? You might eventually get where you want to go, but it would take longer, use more fuel, and probably be pretty frustrating.

3. When a person struggles with sexual arousal, desire, or orgasm, the difficulty might be too little stimulation to the accelerator, or it might be too much stimulation to the brake—and it's usually *too much stimulation to the brake.*

To maximize your sexual wellbeing, notice what activates the accelerator and what hits the brakes, so you can begin shaping your life to turn on the ons and (especially) turn off the offs. In this chapter you'll find several exercises that will help you get to know your sexual brain, both the ways it can be turned on and the ways it can be turned off.

Just as everyone's genitals are made of the same parts,

21

organized in a unique way, everyone has both brakes and an accelerator, but each of us has *different sensitivities* of brakes and accelerator.

Some people are high on both brakes and accelerator, others are low on both brakes and accelerator, some have high brakes but low accelerator, and some have high accelerator but low brakes. And lots of us are medium on both.

You can complete the following questionnaire to get a sense of how sensitive your own brakes and accelerator are. It's adapted and abbreviated from a formal survey used to assess brakes and accelerator in the research, but don't mistake this for actual science. It's intended to guide you in your understanding of how your internal sexual response mechanism may influence your response to sexual stimulation, but it is just an approximation.

sexual temperament questionnaire

(adapted and abbreviated from the Sexual Excitation/Sexual
Inhibition Inventory for Women and Men [SESII-W/M])

Inhibitors

Sometimes I have so many worries that I am unable to get aroused.

0	1	2	3	4
Not at all like me	Not much like me	Somewhat like me	A lot like me	Exactly like me

If I think that I am being used sexually it completely turns me off.

0	1	2	3	4
Not at all like me	Not much like me	Somewhat like me	A lot like me	Exactly like me

If I am uncertain how my partner feels about me, it is harder for me to get aroused.

0	1	2	3	4
Not at all like me	Not much like me	Somewhat like me	A lot like me	Exactly like me

If I am worried about taking too long to become aroused or to orgasm, this can interfere with my arousal.

0	1	2	3	4
Not at all like me	Not much like me	Somewhat like me	A lot like me	Exactly like me

Sometimes I feel so "shy" or self-conscious during sex that I cannot become fully aroused.

0	1	2	3	4
Not at all like me	Not much like me	Somewhat like me	A lot like me	Exactly like me

Total (out of 20) ____

Exciters

Seeing a partner doing something that shows their talent or intelligence, or watching them interacting well with others, can make me very sexually aroused.

0	1	2	3	4
Not at all like me	Not much like me	Somewhat like me	A lot like me	Exactly like me

When I think about someone I find sexually attractive or fantasize about sex, I easily become sexually aroused.

0	1	2	3	4
Not at all like me	Not much like me	Somewhat like me	A lot like me	Exactly like me

If it is possible someone might see or hear us having sex, it is more difficult for me to get aroused.

4	3	2	1	0
Not at all like me	Not much like me	Somewhat like me	A lot like me	Exactly like me

If I am very sexually attracted to someone, I don't need to be in a relationship with that person to become sexually aroused.

0	1	2	3	4
Not at all like me	Not much like me	Somewhat like me	A lot like me	Exactly like me

I think about sex a lot when I am bored.

0	1	2	3	4
Not at all like me	Not much like me	Somewhat like me	A lot like me	Exactly like me

Total (out of 20) ____

score your sexual temperament questionnaire

Inhibitors

Low brakes (0–6)

You're not so sensitive to all the reasons not to be sexually aroused. You don't tend to worry about your own sexual functioning, and body image issues don't interfere too much with your sexuality. When you're sexually engaged, your attention is not very distractible and you wouldn't be inclined to describe yourself as "sexually shy." Most circumstances can be sexual for you. You may find that your main challenge around sexual functioning is holding yourself back. Staying aware of potential consequences can help with this.

Medium brakes (7–13)

You're right in the middle, along with more than half the women I've asked. This means that whether or not your sexual brakes engage will be largely dependent on context. Risky or novel situations, such as a new partner, might increase your concerns about your own sexual functioning, shyness, or your distractibility from sex. Contexts that easily arouse you are likely to be low risk and more familiar, and anytime your stress levels—including anxiety, overwhelm, exhaustion, depression—escalate, your brakes will reduce your interest in and response to sexual signals.

High brakes (14–20)

You're pretty sensitive to all the reasons not to be sexually aroused. You need a setting of trust and relaxation in order to be aroused, and it's best if you don't feel rushed or pressured in any way. You might be easily distracted from sex. High brakes, regardless of accelerator, is the most strongly correlated factor with sexual problems, so if this is you, pay close attention to the "sexy contexts" worksheets in the chapters that follow.

Exciters

Low accelerator (0–6)

You're not so sensitive to sexually relevant stimuli and need to make a more deliberate effort to tune your attention to that wavelength. Novel situations are less likely to be sexy to you than familiar ones. You're a person whose sexual functioning will benefit from adding a greater intensity of stimulation (like a vibrator) and daily practice of paying attention to sensations. Lower accelerator is also associated with asexuality, so if you're very low accelerator, you might resonate with some aspects of the asexual identity.

Medium accelerator (7–13)

You're right in the middle, so whether or not you're sensitive to sexual stimuli probably depends on the context. In situations of high romance or eroticism, you tune in readily to sexual stimuli; and in situations of low romance or eroticism, it may be pretty challenging to move your attention to sexual things. Seventy percent of the women I've asked fall into this range.

High accelerator (14–20)

You're pretty sensitive to sexually relevant stimuli, maybe even things humans aren't generally very sensitive to, like smell and taste. A fairly wide range of contexts can be sexual for you, and novelty may be really exciting. You may be a person who likes having sex as a way to destress—higher accelerator is correlated with greater risk for sexual compulsivity, so you may benefit from paying attention to the ways you manage stress. Your sexual functioning may benefit by making sure you create lots of time and space for your partner; because you're sensitive, you can derive intense satisfaction from your partner's pleasure, so you'll both benefit! About 16 percent of the women I've asked fall into this group.

what "medium" means

Did you score right in the middle on both? More than half of people do. Being very high or very low on these traits is comparatively rare, so for the majority of people, the value of the dual control model lies not in the discovery that, "Wow, my brain is extra sensitive/not sensitive to this kind of stimulation, so I need to pay attention to that!" The value instead lies in the insight that the brakes and the accelerator are *two separate systems*. Some things in the world activate your accelerator, which makes you eager. Other things hit your brakes and slow down your arousal process. Some things hit both at once. Your partner may touch you in a way you really enjoy, but at a time when it's not appropriate for you to be aroused (e.g., in public or when there's risk of unwanted pregnancy).

Every score is "normal." The key is to understand that your brain reacts with both "turning on the ons" and "turning off the offs." Notice what hits your brakes or activates your accelerator, and you can begin to recalibrate your life to suit your brain.

what turns on the ons, what turns off the offs?

Now that you've considered the sensitivities of your brakes and accelerator, let's consider what kinds of stimulation might hit your brakes or activate your accelerator.

Some common things that activate the accelerator: partner characteristics, feeling "wanted" by your partner, feeling connected to your partner, thinking about sex, reading erotica or looking at porn or otherwise consuming sexually explicit media, being touched just the "right" way, being in a setting you associate with sex (e.g., on vacation at a place where you previously had a positive sexual experience).

Some common things that hit the brake: stress, body image, shame, performance anxiety, fear of being interrupted or caught, relationship characteristics (especially trust), a history of sexual trauma, parenting (e.g., constantly being touched by your children, thus associating touch with parenting mode rather than sexy mode), worries about reputation, and feeling expected or obliged to have sex.

Think of a few sexual experiences you've had, whether solo or partnered, and write down what aspects of these experiences activated the accelerator, making it easy to get aroused. And think about times when you've struggled with arousal or desire, and write down what aspects of those experiences hit the brake.

Things that activate the accelerator	Things that hit the brakes

from the q & a vault

Q: **What kind of questions can I ask to learn with my wife what hits her brakes and what hits mine?**

A: The short answer to communication-related questions like this is, just talk about it. Just ask, "What hits your brakes?" The reality, though, is that you may feel like you don't know what words to use or like you should already know the answer or you fear the answer you'll get, or you're worried your partner will judge you for even bringing it up or feel pressured to do something they don't want to do. There are lots of reasons people don't "just talk about it."

Here are a couple of tips to make it easier:

First, ask your partner if now might be a good time to talk about what makes sex good or great between you. If they say no, ask to set up a time when you can talk together, no pressure or expectations, just talk, about what makes sex good or great between you.

Many people find it easiest to begin with the positive stuff. Ask your partner, "When we've had great sex, what was going on in our lives, in our relationship, in that sexual encounter?" People also often find it easier to communicate clearly when they start with a concrete, specific example, rather than trying to talk in general terms.

If you're the one initiating the conversation, be sure to let your partner tell you about what hits their brakes before you talk about what hits yours. If you launch into, "You know what really doesn't work for me . . ." it can too easily feel like a laundry list of complaints, which will just shut the person down or escalate the conversation into an argument. Instead, ask, "What are some things that get in the way of great sex?"

And finally, never end a conversation about sex without

expressing gratitude that you have the kind of relationship where you can talk about these things without judgment or shame or fear. Your sex life together is something you share, like a kid or a mortgage or the chores. It's so easy not to talk about sex, to let your erotic connection dissolve into entropy, so make sure you let your partner know how glad you are they're willing to spend time paying attention to what it takes to make your sexual connection good.

how did you learn?

How do we learn what counts as a "sex-related stimulus"? Are we born being turned on by red high heels or black lace bras? Of course not; these things are learned. Our early experiences with sexual response shape how our body responds to the world.

And that experience is more complex than just "I saw some porn and my body responded." It's more like a toddler learning to walk. When a toddler falls down, her first reaction is to look up at the faces of the adults around her, as though to say, "Something happened! How should I feel about it?" When the adults are calm and chirp, "You fell down. You're okay!" the toddler gets back up and keeps going. But if the adults panic and run over, exclaiming, "Be careful, you could get hurt!" the toddler panics, too, and bursts into tears.

In the same way, you learn what's "sex-related" not just because your genitals respond to something, but because you noticed your *environment*, especially the other people there with you in the situation.

So in this exercise, you'll note as many experiences of sexual learning as you can recall, beginning with your earliest memories. This can include:

- Formal education in a classroom setting. .
- Explicit sexual messages you received elsewhere.
- Porn and other sexually explicit media.
- Implicit sexual messages, such as messages about what clothes were appropriate.

- Solo sexual experiences.
- Sexual experiences with others.

You might want to organize this history of sexual learning in terms of what trained your accelerator and what trained your brake, or you might find that too many of your experiences were ambivalent, teaching both at the same time. You may prefer to make a straightforward list or chronology.

Take your time with this, and know that you can come back as you remember more experiences. This history will form the beginning of your "sexual mental model," and we'll come back to it in more detail in later chapters. Include specific incidents, conversations, and feelings you remember experiencing as these moments happened. For example, if a family member gave you "the talk," include how you felt at the time, how you imagine they felt, how you feel now as you remember it, and how that conversation affected you later.

Birth through childhood—your earliest memories of sex. Were you curious about sex? What sexual play did you engage in as a child? How did that feel for you? Were the other people involved your peers (other children) or not? How did the adults around you respond, if they knew about it?

Puberty through adolescence—your development toward sexual adulthood. When did you first see porn, and how did you feel about it? What kinds of porn have you been accidentally exposed to, and what have you sought? Did you first masturbate during this stage? Where? And how? How did you feel about it? If you were ever "caught," how did that experience feel?

Adulthood through the present—the sexual person you are and the person you're "supposed" to be. What have been some defining moments in your development as a sexual adult? When has it been a source of joy and pleasure in your life? Have you ever felt out of control in your sexuality? This might be compulsive masturbation, persistent arousal, or seeking partners you didn't really want or like but simply felt compelled, from an internal discomfort, to seek out sex. Or it might be an experience where someone else took away your control over your body or you were coerced into things you didn't want or like.

The exercises from this chapter will inform many of the exercises in the coming chapters, so feel free to come back and add to or change them as you learn more about your sexuality.

one important thing

Take a moment to look back at the exercises in this chapter. Write down one important thing you learned, whether it's about sex in general or about your sexuality in particular:

three

context

In chapter 2, we talked about sex-related stimuli as sensations and perceptions that your brain learned to associate with sexual arousal. But it's more complicated than just "this turns me on" and "that turns me off." A sensation, thought, or image that turns us on in a sex-positive setting might be actively unpleasant in a different setting.

The most obvious example of this difference between sensation and perception is tickling. Not everyone loves to be tickled, but at least hypothetically you can imagine a situation where you're in a flirty, playful, sexy state of mind, and your certain special someone tickles you. In that context, the tickling might be pleasurable and lead to further play. But if that same certain special someone tries to tickle you when you're angry with them, how does that feel?

Like maybe you want to punch them in the face.

Whether a sensation is perceived as pleasurable or uncomfortable depends on the context in which we perceive it. This is not because of conscious, intentional choice. The change in perception begins at a fundamental level, down in the emotional parts of the brain. When you're in a great, sex-positive context, almost everything can activate your curious, desirous approach to sex. And when you're in a not-so-great, stressful context— whether due to external circumstances or internal factors like self-criticism or performance anxiety—it doesn't matter how sexy your partner is, how much you love them, or how fancy your underwear is, almost nothing will activate that curious, exploring, desirous experience.

what does a sex-positive context look like?

So what counts as a sex-positive context, according to science?

In general, a person's brain is most likely to interpret the world as a safe, fun, sexy, pleasurable place when the context is:

High trust, high affection, low stress, and explicitly erotic.

More specifically, a great, sex-positive context means:

- *Mental and physical wellbeing:* Being confident and healthy, both emotionally and physically, without undue stress or pain.
- *Partner characteristics:* Having an attractive partner who respects you and accepts you as you are.
- *Relationship characteristics:* Feeling trusting and affectionate in your relationship; feeling desired by your partner.
- *Setting:* Being in a setting that lets the "offs" turn off and the "ons" turn on—perhaps on vacation or perhaps at home with the door locked—and being approached in a way that makes

you feel special; explicitly erotic cues, like erotica or porn, or hearing or seeing other people having sex.

- *Other life circumstances:* Life stressors, family, work, money, the state of the world, and all the other nonsexual factors that influence the state of our brains.
- *Ludic factors:* "Ludic," coming from the same word origin as "ludicrous," means "play." Do you feel free to experiment, explore, and play with your partner? What sexual things do you *enjoy* doing?

consider the context

In this first exercise, you'll think through what contexts work for you. You'll think of three great sexual experiences you've had, then three not-so-great ones—not terrible, just sort of okay. You'll consider the relevant aspects of the context and identify which aspects increased or diminished the pleasure of that experience.

It may seem like a lot to think carefully about six different sexual experiences. You can start with one of each, but the more experiences you can compare and contrast, the more insight you'll get. You'll start to see patterns that weren't apparent until you examined in this systematic way what about these contexts shaped the readiness of your brain to interpret the world as a safe, fun, sexy, pleasurable place.

sexy context #1

Think of a positive sexual experience from your past. Describe it here, with as many relevant details as you can recall, including where you were, whom you were with, how you felt about each other on that day, the health and wellbeing of each partner, and the outside life circumstances that may have influenced your state of mind:

Looking at what you wrote, mark the places where you refer to any of these six factors that influence context. (You may choose to use different styles of marking—underlining, circling, an asterisk, and so on, or you may prefer to use different-color highlighters or simply write, for example, "partner characteristics" in the margin.)

1. *Mental and physical wellbeing:* Physical health/body image, mood/anxiety, distractibility, worry about sexual functioning

2. *Partner characteristics:* Physical appearance, physical health, smell, mental state

3. *Relationship characteristics:* Trust, power dynamic, emotional connection, feeling desired, frequency of sex

4. *Setting:* Private/public, home, work, vacation, etc.; distance sex (phone, online chat, etc.); see partner do something positive, like interact with family or do work

5. *Other life circumstances:* Work-related stress, family-related stress, holiday, anniversary, other occasion

6. *Ludic factors:* Self-guided fantasy, partner-guided fantasy (talking dirty), body parts that were touched or not, oral sex on you/on partner, intercourse, etc.

sexy context #2

Think of a positive sexual experience from your past. Describe it here in a few sentences:

```
┌─────────────────────────────────────────────┐
│                                             │
│                                             │
│                                             │
│                                             │
│                                             │
└─────────────────────────────────────────────┘
```

With that experience in mind, consider what aspects of that experience made it positive:

Category	Description
Mental and physical wellbeing: Physical health/ body image, mood/ anxiety, distractibility, worry about sexual functioning	
Partner characteristics: Physical appearance, physical health, smell, mental state	
Relationship characteristics: Trust, power dynamic, emotional connection, feeling desired, frequency of sex	

Category	Description
Setting: Private/public, home, work, vacation, etc.; distance sex (phone, online chat, etc.); see partner do something positive, like interact with family or do work	
Other life circumstances: Work-related stress, family-related stress, holiday, anniversary, other occasion	
Ludic factors: Self-guided fantasy, partner-guided fantasy (talking dirty), body parts that were touched or not, oral sex on you/on partner, intercourse, etc.	
Other:	

sexy context #3

By now you may be getting a sense of which aspects of context are key to making a sexual experience great, whether it's your own wellbeing, partner characteristics, relationship characteristics, setting, other life circumstances, or what you actually do during sex. If one or two factors stand out as key, circle them here:

key contextual factor (circle one or two)

My physical and mental wellbeing   Other life circumstances

Partner characteristics   Ludic factors

Relationship characteristics   Other: _____

Setting

Describe another great sexual experience where the key factor was strong, with as many relevant details as you can recall:

Now consider what aspects the context *amplified* the key factor you chose. Just as you did in the first worksheet of this exercise, mark the places where you refer to any of these other factors. (Again, you may choose to use different styles of marking— underlining, circling, an asterisk, and so on, or you may prefer to use different-color highlighters, or simply write, for example, "partner characteristics" in the margin.)

Finally, in the margins of what you wrote, write a sentence or two about how different factors amplified the key factor. For example, if your key factor is "relationship characteristics" and the great sex happened when your partner came in from mowing the lawn, the key factor of the relationship could have been amplified by the partner characteristic of their smell. Or if your key factor is "mental and physical wellbeing" and the great sex happened while you were on vacation, some details about that vacation may have amplified your sense of wellbeing.

not-so-sexy context #1

Think of a not-so-great sexual experience from your past—not a terrible one, just a mediocre or mildly disappointing one. Describe it here, with as many relevant details as you can recall, including where you were, whom you were with, how you felt about each other on that day, the health and wellbeing of each partner, and the outside life circumstances that may have influenced your state of mind:

Looking at what you wrote, mark the places where you refer to any of these six factors that influence context. (You may choose to use different styles of marking—underlining, circling, an asterisk, and so on, or you may prefer to use different-color highlighters, or simply write, for example, "partner characteristics" in the margin.)

1. *Mental and physical wellbeing:* Physical health/body image, mood/anxiety, distractibility, worry about sexual functioning

2. *Partner characteristics:* Physical appearance, physical health, smell, mental state

3. *Relationship characteristics:* Trust, power dynamic, emotional connection, feeling desired, frequency of sex

4. *Setting:* Private/public, home, work, vacation, etc.; distance sex (phone, online chat, etc.); see partner do something positive, like interact with family or do work

5. *Other life circumstances:* Work-related stress, family-related stress, holiday, anniversary, other occasion

6. *Ludic factors:* Self-guided fantasy, partner-guided fantasy (talking dirty), body parts that were touched or not, oral sex on you/on partner, intercourse, etc.

not-so-sexy context #2

Think of another not-so-great sexual experience from your past. Describe it here in a few sentences:

With that experience in mind, consider what aspects of that experience made it not so great:

Category	Description
Mental and physical wellbeing: Physical health/ body image, mood/ anxiety, distractibility, worry about sexual functioning	
Partner characteristics: Physical appearance, physical health, smell, mental state	
Relationship characteristics: Trust, power dynamic, emotional connection, feeling desired, frequency of sex	

Category	Description
Setting: Private/public, home, work, vacation etc.; distance sex (phone, online chat, etc.); see partner do something positive, like interact with family or do work	
Other life circumstances: Work-related stress, family-related stress, holiday, anniversary, other occasion	
Ludic factors: Self-guided fantasy, partner-guided fantasy (talking dirty), body parts that were touched or not, oral sex on you/on partner, intercourse, etc.	
Other:	

not-so-sexy context #3

By now you may be getting a sense of which aspects of context are key to making a sexual experience not so great, whether it's your own wellbeing, partner characteristics, relationship characteristics, setting, other life circumstances, or what you actually do during sex. If one or two factors stand out as key, circle them here:

key contextual factor (circle one or two)

My physical and mental wellbeing   Other life circumstances

Partner characteristics   Ludic factors

Relationship characteristics   Other: _____

Setting

Describe another not-so-great sexual experience where the key factor was strong, with as many relevant details as you can recall:

Now consider what aspects the context *amplified* the key factor you chose. Just as you did in the previous worksheet, mark the places where you refer to any of these other factors. (Once again, you may choose to use different styles of marking—underlining, circling, an asterisk, and so on, or you may prefer to use different-color highlighters, or simply write, for example, "partner characteristics" in the margin.)

Finally, in the margins of what you wrote, write a sentence or two about how different factors amplified the key factor. For example, if your key factor is "relationship characteristics" and the not-so-great sex happened when you felt obliged to have sex even though you were feeling disconnected from your partner, the key factor of the relationship could have been amplified by your mental and physical wellbeing. Or if your key factor is "mental and physical wellbeing" and the not-so-great sex happened while you were on vacation, some details about that vacation may have amplified your sense of a *lack* of wellbeing.

Once you've taken the time to think carefully about your past experiences, you'll find patterns and insights into how context influences your sexual wellbeing. In the next exercise, you'll look more closely at these patterns.

assess the context

Read through all your sexy and not-so-sexy contexts from exercise one. What do you notice as reliable contexts for great sex, and reliable contexts for not-so-great sex? (Reminder: many people find the most sex-positive contexts are low stress, high trust, high affection, and explicitly erotic—but people vary! We're all made of the same parts, but those parts are organized in different ways.)

Contexts That Make Sex Great	Contexts That Make Sex Not So Great

Let's get a little more detailed with this list.

- Not all contextual factors are equally impactful. Draw a ★ or ❤ or other mark next to the great factors that feel most important in creating a sex-positive context for you.
- Draw an X or a ☹ or other mark next to the not-so-great

factors that feel most important in creating a sex-negative context for you.

- Circle or underline or highlight to mark the great factors that you have access to on a regular basis.
- Mark the not-so-great factors you have access to on a regular basis.

When you look at this list of contextual factors that make sex great or not so great, what do you notice? For example, of the great factors, how many are part of your day-to-day life? How many of the important, starred factors are there? How about the not-so-great factors?

from the q & a vault

Q: I learned that the context that kills my sex drive is feeling like I'm required to have sex, and I don't see any way to change that.

A: Remember, the goal is to change the context, not to change how you feel. How you feel will change when you change the context.

So look at the contexts that make you feel like you're "required" to have sex. What's going on in your personal wellbeing? What's happening with your partner? With your relationship? The setting? Other life factors? Is it when you're on vacation and you feel like this is your one chance to have sex without the kids interrupting? Is it when your partner has been hinting or outright asking and you've been too stressed or distracted to say yes, but you're starting to feel bad about always saying no?

No one is ever required to have sex. No matter how much you want to satisfy your partner, no matter how much your partner feels sad about your lack of desire, no matter how much sex you think you're "supposed" to be having, no one is ever required to have sex.

In fact, I'm going to suggest that you take sex entirely off the menu temporarily.

There are fuller instructions on how to implement a change like this in chapter 7 of *CAYA*, but the short explanation is: you are not allowed to touch your own or each other's genitals in the other person's presence until you experience a context where you don't feel required to have sex—which will be easier than you would think, once you've created a context where you're required *not* to have sex.

how to create change

When people struggle with their sexuality or notice changes that trouble them, it's rarely because there's something wrong with them. It's much more likely something in their context has changed, whether it's personal wellbeing, partner characteristics, relationship factors, or life circumstances that have nothing to do with sex. That means that when you consider creating change, often it's more effective to focus on changing the context than on changing *you*.

You can think of the factors you listed under "Contexts That Make Sex Great" in exercise 2 as your ideal sexual context. Of course, life is rarely ideal! But what if you could change your context, to make it just a little better?

This is the first chapter where you'll begin to explore intentional ways to create change in your sexuality. The change-based worksheets in this book all follow a similar format, designed to help you consider what you might do if you decided to try something new. This includes thinking through the concrete, specific steps you might take, anticipating the barriers that might arise, and asking yourself how important this step is and how confident you feel that you could make it happen, if you chose to.

The "if you chose" matters. Thinking about what it would take to create change *does not commit you to creating change*! If you are ambivalent about change, that's normal, and in fact thinking through what steps you might take can help to resolve your ambivalence one way or the other. You may also discover that many of the factors influencing your context are not in your control, which can be liberating, because it shows you what you can let go. Accepting the uncontrollable factors allows you to have realistic expectations about just how sex-positive your life can be or can't be right now.

This process of (1) identifying an impactful-yet-doable strategy; (2) making a concrete, specific plan for implementing it; (3) anticipating barriers; and (4) assessing and maximizing motivation and confidence is an evidence-based approach to creating changes of all kinds, from having better sex to quitting smoking to changing careers. Use it whenever you want to create change and are feeling stuck.

hypothetical change

Brainstorm a dozen (or more!) changes you and/or your partner could hypothetically make if you decided to work toward creating more frequent and easier access to the contexts that make sex great. (Tip: getting rid of things that hit the brakes can be more important than adding stimulation to the accelerator.)

1. _____
2. _____
3. _____
4. _____
5. _____
6. _____
7. _____
8. _____
9. _____
10. _____
11. _____
12. _____
More: _____

Select six of these ideas and consider:

1. *how impactful* you expect them to be (use the marking system you used in the previous worksheet, whether hearts or frowny faces or a zero-to-ten scale, and so on, to indicate their impact)

2. *how easy* they would be to implement

3. *how soon* you can do them

A silly example, to illustrate: "Not having kids" might have a huge impact on your context—nine out of ten hearts!—but that kind of change is neither easy (parenting: possibly the most difficult thing you'll ever do) nor immediate (like maybe ten years from now, when the youngest goes to college). Putting on socks, though, is easy, quick, and can make a surprising difference! In fact, putting on socks made it easier for research participants to orgasm while masturbating in a brain imaging machine. Why? According to the researcher leading the study, the research participants "were uncomfortable because they had cold feet." Put on socks, have warmer feet, release the brake, and have easier orgasms. So if your strategy is "warm feet," you expect it to be a little bit impactful— four out of ten hearts—but it's easy (you put on socks almost every day) and you can do it right now.

Or maybe "feeling obligated to have sex" is a factor that hits the brakes. How impactful would it be to eliminate the feeling of obligation? Twelve out of ten hearts! How easy would it be? *Oh, boy*, you think, *I wouldn't even know where to start*. And how soon could you do it? As soon as you figured out what to do, probably.

Don't worry if you don't currently know what to do to create change. That's the next worksheet.

Right now, choose six of your hypothetical change strategies.

Then set a timer for six minutes—that's one minute per strategy, to prevent yourself from getting bogged down in details—and assess each strategy's potential impact, easiness, and how soon you could apply it.

	Change	How much impact?	How easy?	How soon can you do it?
1				
2				
3				
4				
5				
6				

By this point, you might be feeling supermotivated and ready to create change. Or you might be feeling bored or overwhelmed and want to quit and do something else, anything else, to avoid having to think systematically about creating change. (So many boxes! Please, no more boxes!)

Planning for change is painstaking. This step-by-step process is the most evidence-based way to create change, but I call it painstaking for a reason. You did not get to the place you're in now by accident. It took years of practice—sometimes intentional, sometimes not—to get where you are, so change will not always be instantaneous or easy.

If you ever feel overwhelmed, discouraged, or disengaged in this process, recruit a friend, partner, therapist, or coach to work with you. Or you might decide that now is not the time for change. Skip to exercise 5, "Motivation for Change," if you're wondering if the effort it takes to create change is worthwhile.

planning for change

There are lots of ways to imagine the path from where you are to where you want to be. Here are a few you can try:

1. **Planful problem-solving.** Ask yourself, "If I decide to create this change, what goes on the to-do list?"
2. **Reverse engineering.** Imagine what it will be like after you've implemented the strategy, and then think backward. What did you do to get there?
3. **Strengths-based.** You've made changes in the past. What strengths do you bring to the table that allowed you to make that change?

Select one or maybe two of your top change ideas that feel like the right combination of impact, ease, and immediacy, and identify what would have to happen for them to become reality. Be as *concrete* and *specific* as you can. These should be *actions*, rather than abstractions or ideas or attitudes. In the space below, describe a hypothetical action plan for a change you selected, including a start date.

Name of Plan (e.g., "Operation Sexypants"): _____

Start Date: _____

Description of Plan:

What behavioral, emotional, physical, or interpersonal change will show you your plan is working?

Finally, anticipate the likely barriers that might prevent you from being able to follow through on your plan, and choose a strategy for handling that barrier should it arise. For example, if you're eliminating the feeling of obligation to have sex and your plan includes discussing it with your partner, a potential barrier might be, "My partner says or does something to affirm they do feel I'm obliged to have sex," and your strategy for handling it might be, "Remind them that our goal with the conversation is to improve our sex life and that the feeling of obligation is hitting my brakes, so I'm asking for their help in eliminating that sense of obligation."

Likely Barrier	Strategy for Handling It

motivation for change

Now that you've thought through what you might do if you decided to create change, let's consider how important change is to you and why.

Considering the plan you made in the previous exercise, ask yourself these questions:

On a scale of zero to ten, how *important* would you say it is for you to make this change?

0	1	2	3	4	5	6	7	8	9	10

What makes it that important and not a zero (or two or four, etc.)?

On a scale of zero to ten, how *confident* would you say you are that you could make this change if you decided you wanted to?

0	1	2	3	4	5	6	7	8	9	10

What makes it not a zero (or two or four, etc.)? What past experience do you have that tells you your strategy could work?

Sometimes creating change is fun and easy, but sometimes it's exhausting and can even make you feel helpless or isolated. If that happens, call on your support network. Sharing your process with a friend can make all the difference.

So far in the workbook you've thought about the basic hardware of your sexuality—your body, your brain, and the context in which they function. In the next section, we're going to take a closer look at context and how you can shape your life and your world to maximize your sexual wellbeing.

one important thing

Take a moment to look back at the exercises in this chapter. Write down one important thing you learned, whether it's about sex in general or about your sexuality in particular:

part two

sex in context

four

emotional context

We know that context influences whether and when our brains are ready to interpret any sensation as sexy. We even have a sense of what contexts facilitate our brain's perception of the world as a safe, fun, sexy, pleasurable place.

Now what?

Now we delve into one specific aspect of context that almost universally influences our perception of sex-related sensations: *stress*. As we mentioned in chapters 2 and 3, stress can hit the brakes for a lot of people. It's easy to understand why; stress is a biological reaction that alters your physiology, including brain functioning, to let you know your body is not safe right now. And of course if you're not safe, it may not be a good time to have sex.

To reduce the impact of stress on your sexual pleasure and interest, to have more joyful, pleasurable sex, manage your stress.

"Sure, Emily," you say. "Manage my stress. Like it's that easy."
Sometimes it's not easy. But it is definitely doable!

In the worksheets that follow, you'll practice genuinely effective, evidence-based approaches to addressing stress so it can get out of the way of your sex life.

from the q & a vault

Q: My partner and I are both very stressed at times, but when I'm stressed my sex drive goes through the roof, but my partner's seems to disappear. What do we do? Is there something wrong with one of us?

A: Nope, there is nothing wrong with either of you. People vary— all the same parts, organized in different ways. Roughly 10 to 20 percent of people may experience an increase in sexual interest when they experience stress, depression, anxiety, or other uncomfortable emotions. The rest experience either no change or a reduction in their interest in sex. All those variations are normal. And even for the 10 to 20 percent, stress blocks sexual pleasure even as it increases sexual interest. Stressed sex feels different from joyful sex because: context.

It can be a challenge to manage this kind of discrepancy in a relationship, but when you know that both people are normal, that neither is "wrong," you can begin to collaborate to create a sexuality that works for both of you. You can compromise. Maybe you can ask the lower-desire partner to watch while you masturbate. Maybe you can support your partner in reducing their stress level enough to free up their brake so they can be interested in sex. Maybe just knowing neither of you is broken can reduce your stress enough to reduce the feeling of urgency in your desire for sex. And probably your relationship is strong enough to withstand the temporary waves of stress that life brings, knowing that you'll be able to reconnect when life becomes more stable.

exercise one

separating stress from the stressors

Brainstorm the brakes-hitting stressors in your life—things you
worry about, things you have to do "or else," and things that ex-
haust or overwhelm you. Write down at least a dozen (though there
are likely more). Get it all off your chest:

1. _____
2. _____
3. _____
4. _____
5. _____
6. _____
7. _____
8. _____
9. _____
10. _____
11. _____
12. _____

Look at your list of stressors and draw a line through those you
mostly can't control in the immediate future—like having children
and/or a job, struggling financially, or being in a bad living situation.

Then circle the stressors that you could do something about in
the short term. We'll call these "controllable stressors." Take a moment to list the three controllable stressors that have a significant
impact on your sexuality.

top controllable stressors

1. _____

2. _____

3. _____

If you're looking for ways to manage these controllable stressors, great! Use exercises 3, 4, and 5—"Hypothetical Change," "Planning for Change," and "Motivation for Change"—from chapter 3 to create a plan. If you're not, that's also great! It's up to you. Either way, always remember that the plan you make to deal with your *stressors* is a separate thing from the plan you make to deal with *the stress itself*. That's the next exercise.

recognizing your stress

For this worksheet, you'll turn your attention inward, to notice how stress manifests in your body.

Think of a time when you felt obviously stressed. Take a moment to describe the circumstances here:

Now, remembering how it felt to be stressed in those circumstances, identify the signs of stress in your body, emotions, and thoughts:

Physical Signs of Stress (e.g., digestive upset, jaw tension, etc.)	Emotional Signs of Stress (e.g., tearful, easily frustrated, etc.)	Cognitive Signs of Stress (e.g., distracted, unfocused, etc.)

This is your stress. It's important to know what stress feels like, so you can recognize when it is gone.

recognizing relaxation

For this worksheet, notice how safety and calm manifest in your body.

Think of a time when you felt safe and relieved of your stress—regardless of whether you'd been relieved of the *cause* of the stress. Take a moment to describe the circumstances here:

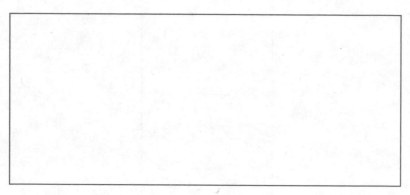

Now, remembering how it felt to be calm and safe in those circumstances, identify the signs of safety and calm in your body, emotions, and thoughts:

Physical Signs of Calm (e.g., muscles, digestion, facial tension)	Emotional Signs of Calm (e.g., laughing readily, slow to frustrate, loving)	Cognitive Signs of Calm (e.g., focused, logical, shifting attention at will)

Next, we'll look at how you got to that state of relaxation.

complete the cycle

Once you've identified your stress and what causes it, the next step is to complete the *stress response cycle*, so your body can shift from "Your body is not safe right now" to "Your body is a safe place to be."

In the environment where humans evolved, the behaviors that eliminated the stress in our bodies were the behaviors that eliminated the stressors out in the world. If we ran away from the lion that was chasing us, we escaped the lion.

These days, we are almost never chased by lions, but your body's reactions to modern stressors is basically the same; whether it's traffic or your kids who won't put on their shoes or the state of world politics, your body's response is adrenaline and cortisol, increased blood pressure, and reduced cognitive flexibility. And getting out of traffic or convincing your child to put on their shoes or changing world politics may deal with the stressor . . . but that doesn't mean you dealt with the stress. You get out of traffic and you're still carrying the tension in your shoulders or lower back, and your emotions are still making you feel like you want to stab someone. Your kid puts on their shoes, and your jaw is still tense, your stomach is in knots, and your thoughts are still focused on the frustrations of parenting.

Why is it that we can deal with a stressor and yet not deal with the stress? Because your body doesn't know what "out of traffic" means; it doesn't know what "patiently stand over child until shoes are on feet" means. Neither of these are part of the evolutionary mechanism designed to help us escape predators.

When you're being chased by a lion, what do you do?

You run.

The running itself, not the elimination of the lion, is what shifts your physiology out of "Your body is not safe right now" into "Your body is a safe place to be."

So when you're stressed out by your job or your family or even by your sex life, what do you do?

You run . . . or walk, or get on the elliptical machine or go out dancing or even just dance around your bedroom. *Moving your body* is the single most efficient strategy for completing the stress response cycle and recalibrating your central nervous system into a calm state. When people say, "Exercise is good for stress," this is a big part of why. Exercise is not the only way, of course; it's just arguably the most efficient.

Here are some other things that science says can genuinely help us not only feel better but actually facilitate the completion of the stress response cycle:

- Sleep.
- Affection.
- Any form of meditation, including mindfulness, yoga, tai chi, body scans, and so on.
- A big ol' cry or primal scream—though you have to be careful with this one. Sometimes people just wallow in their stress when they cry, rather than allowing the tears to wash away the stress. If you've had the experience of locking yourself in your room and sobbing for ten minutes, and then at the end heaving a great big sigh and feeling tremendously relieved, you've felt how it can move you through the stress response cycle.

- Any form of art or creative self-expression. When mental health professionals suggest journaling or other expressive self-care, they don't mean that the construction of sentences or the task of drawing is inherently therapeutic; rather, they're encouraging you to find positive contexts to discharge your stress, through the creative process.

what completes the cycle?

Remember that moment when you felt relaxed, safe, and calm? What did you do to help that happen? This isn't about the stressor going away; it's about your body transitioning through the cycle. Identify any evidence-based practices that were helpful, or name your own:

what helps complete the cycle

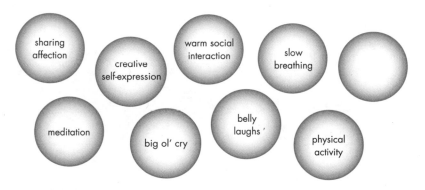

Here you'll write your go-to plan whenever you're experiencing overwhelming stress.

> When I'm feeling stressed, overwhelmed, or exhausted, here's what helps:

considering change

Of the things you just identified, choose one (for now) to think about what it would take to increase your access to it. Suppose, hypothetically, you decided you wanted to use this stress management strategy more. What might be some challenges you'd face if you tried to use it more? If you've tried in the past to use this strategy, what got in your way?

What are some things you might do to minimize those barriers if you decided to try using this stress management strategy more?

On a scale of zero to ten, how *important* would you say it is for you to make this change?

0	1	2	3	4	5	6	7	8	9	10

What makes it that important and not a zero (or two or four, etc.)?

On a scale of zero to ten, how *confident* would you say you are that you could make this change if you decided you wanted to?

0	1	2	3	4	5	6	7	8	9	10

What makes it not a zero (or two or four, etc.)? What past experience do you have that tells you your strategy could work?

Given all of that, what's one thing you could try *today* to move just one step closer to being able to use this stress management strategy more? (You can always go back to the "creating change" worksheets if you want to make a concrete, specific plan.)

when sex is the lion: sexual trauma

Beyond the day-to-day stresses of life, sometimes there are deep wounds that life inflicts and does not always provide opportunities to heal. Sexual trauma is highly prevalent—a conservative estimate is that about a quarter of women experience sexual violence in their lifetime—so it's impossible to talk about women's sexual health without spending some time discussing trauma. From childhood sexual abuse to sexual assault to all forms of intimate partner violence, women are disproportionately and systematically targeted, and thus they disproportionately bring to their sexual functioning the emotional, physical, and cognitive features of a trauma survivor.

Trauma happens when a person's control over their body is taken from them. Whether the cause is a car accident or sexual violence, the survival mechanism kicks in: freeze, a petrified shutdown characterized by numbness and sometimes immobility or a sense of disembodiment. There is no "fight" response, because the threat is too immediate and inescapable. Sometimes people describe it as "going into shock."

Trauma isn't always caused by a specific incident. It can also emerge in response to persistent distress or ongoing abuse, like a relationship where sex is unwanted, though it may be technically "consensual" because the targeted person says yes in order to avoid being hurt, or they feel trapped in the relationship or are otherwise coerced. In that context, a survivor's body gradually learns that it can't escape and it can't fight; freeze becomes the default stress response because of the learned pattern of shutdown as the best way to guarantee survival.

Sexual violence often doesn't look like "violence," as we usually imagine it—rarely is there a gun or knife or even "aggression"

89

as we typically think of it. Instead, there is coercion and the removal of a person's choice about what will happen next.

Sexual trauma survivorship impacts both the accelerator and the brake. Sensations, contexts, and ideas that used to be interpreted as "sex-related" may instead now be interpreted by your brain as threats, so that sexy contexts actually hit the brakes. And the chronically high levels of stress activity in a recovering survivor's brain can block out sexual stimuli.

There are three broad approaches to coping with residual trauma: "top-down," or a cognitive, thought-based approach like cognitive behavioral therapy or dialectical behavior therapy; "bottom-up," or a somatic, body-based approach like Sensorimotor Psychotherapy; and a "sideways," mindfulness-based approach. All three can be done with a therapist or other professional provider, and an Internet search of any of these treatment modalities will show you more in-depth information.

What all three approaches share is the creation of a nonreactive awareness of your internal experience, whether thoughts, emotions, or physical sensations. Essentially, you are getting out of your body's way and witnessing it as it does what it does intuitively, which is heal.

nonjudgmental attention

Mindfulness meditations are among the most evidence-based interventions for treating sexual difficulties as diverse as sexual pain, desire difficulties, and orgasm issues, as well as trauma.

Mindfulness is the practice of nonjudgmental, present-centered awareness, neutrally noticing what's happening in the here and now. It is about both *what* you pay attention to—that is, the present moment—and *how* you pay attention to it, with curiosity, openness, and acceptance. Nonjudgment, the "active ingredient" in mindfulness, is not sitting still or noticing your breath or being aware of your senses; it is the *nonjudgment* of whatever you're aware of.

If you're interested in exploring how mindfulness can improve your sex life, even when you're recovering from trauma, *Better Sex through Mindfulness* by Lori Brotto is for you. But here's the short version of how to practice mindfulness:

Start with two minutes. For two minutes a day, direct your attention to your breath as the air comes into your body and your chest and belly expand, and as the breath leaves your body and your chest and belly deflate.

The first thing that will happen is your mind will wander to something else. That's normal. That's healthy. In fact, that's the point! Notice that your mind wandered, let those extraneous thoughts go—you can return to them as soon as the two minutes are up—and allow your attention to return to your breath.

This regular two-minute practice will gradually result in periodic moments throughout the day when you notice what you're paying attention to and then decide if that's what you want to pay attention to right now, or if you want to focus on something else. That's part of the power of mindfulness—it lets you be in control of your brain, so your brain isn't in control of you. But *what* you pay attention to matters less than *how* you pay attention.

one important thing

Take a moment to look back at the exercises in this chapter. Write down one important thing you learned, whether it's about sex in general or your sexuality in particular:

five

cultural context

A woman approached me after a workshop to ask about orgasm. She wanted to know why she wasn't having them during sex.

"Tell me what you mean by sex," I said.

"Um, you know . . ." she said. "When he puts his . . . in my . . ."

"Penile vaginal intercourse?" I asked, and she nodded gratefully.

"Do you have orgasms from other stimulation?"

She said yes.

I let her know that less than a third of women are reliably orgasmic with vaginal penetration; the remaining two-thirds are sometimes, rarely, or never orgasmic from that kind of stimulation, for the simple reason that vaginal stimulation is often an inefficient way to stimulate the clitoris.

Her face changed, the worry melting away at the wonderment of this news.

"You're saying I'm normal?" she said.

Yup.

That small piece of information was transformational. Her and her partner's shame at not being able to do it "right" had acted as a wall that had grown between them, but with one little fact, the wall began to crumble.

Humans create rules about what sex is "right" or "wrong," "good" or "bad." Then we worry about whether we're following them and we judge others if they don't. And yet almost none of those rules have anything to do with how human sexuality really works, since the way it really works is simply "people vary."

In this chapter, you'll explore the rules you've learned about sex that are causing the worry, examine the sources, and begin to consider which of those lessons you'd like to keep and which you'd rather discard. It's a kind of "life-changing magic" tidying of your sexual beliefs and attitudes. In *The Life-Changing Magic of Tidying Up*, Marie Kondo tells us to hold each object we own up to our hearts and ask ourselves, "Does this spark joy?" If it does, we keep it. If not, we discard it, giving grateful thanks to that object for the service it performed while it was with us.

It's time to get our sexual houses in order, so that can we live surrounded only by what contributes to pleasure in our lives.

the "ideal" sexual woman

In this activity you'll examine the messages you've absorbed about how the "ideal" sexual woman looks and behaves. It may help to refer to the "How Did You Learn?" exercise in chapter 2.

We receive messages about the ideal sexual woman from a variety of sources, whose ideas about "ideal" may or may not align. Let's consider three of them:

Moral Messages: Religious and spiritual messages coming either directly from your religious group or more implicitly through ideas of "purity" and "goodness." When you think of a "pure" or "good" sexual woman, what is she like?

To begin, let's give her a name: _____

What does this ideal, "pure" woman look like, and how does she behave outside sexual situations?

How does she initiate sex, if she does?

What does she do and how does she feel during sex?

How does her partner feel about her sexuality?

What would she *never* do or experience?

[ ]

Medical Messages: What we receive from our doctors and our formal sex education (if we have any) and news about medical treatments related to sexual health, such as medication for erectile dysfunction and hormones for menopause. When you imagine a sexually "healthy" or "normal" woman, as defined by the medical profession or scientists, what is she like?

Her name is: _____

What does this ideal healthy, normal woman look like, and how does she behave outside sexual situations?

[ ]

How does she initiate sex, if she does?

What does she do and how does she feel during sex?

How does her partner feel about her sexuality?

What would she *never* do or experience?

Media Messages: This includes television and movies, magazines and books, all forms of pop culture. These are often messages not about "purity" or "health," but about *performance*—all seventy-four types of orgasms you should be having and forty-two tricks to make his dick happy. When you imagine the ideal sexual woman, sprung to life from the pages of the magazine rack in a drugstore or manifested by a spell from the union of television and porn, what is she like?

Her name is: _____

What does this ideal, "peak-performance" woman look like, and how does she behave outside sexual situations?

How does she initiate sex, if she does?

What does she do and how does she feel during sex?

How does her partner feel about her sexuality?

What would she *never* do or experience?

your sexual model

Together, our three versions of the ideal woman constitute a *sexual mental model*, a standard by which each of us, unconsciously or consciously, assesses our own sexuality, to decide whether we're doing it right. When you see yours together, some patterns might emerge. Let's investigate further.

Step 1. Highlight, underline, or circle the characteristics shared by all three. Star or mark any characteristic that is unique to just one of them. Do any of those unique characteristics contradict each other?

Step 2. When you think about what "normal" sex looks like and whether you are normal, which ideal (or which aspects of different ideals) sets the standard against which you assess your own sexuality? Why that one?

Step 3. What are the consequences, both real and imagined, for not conforming with the ideal?

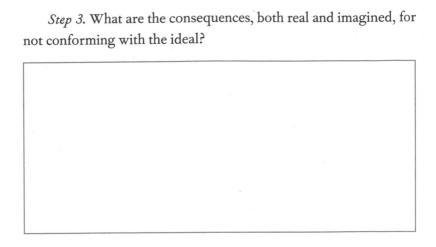

It's important to remember that just as there is no right or wrong sexuality, only the reality that people vary, there is no right or wrong sexual model. Most of us didn't get to choose the messages we were exposed to early in our lives, so our sexual model isn't something we chose. In the next exercise, we'll explore what aspects of your unique sexual model you'd like to keep and which you'd like to discard.

"sex-positive world"

From the beginning of the written record, humanity has had rules about what "right" sex is, and those rules have been as varied as they could possibly be. We've had monogamous cultures, polygynous cultures (one man, multiple women), polyandrous cultures (one woman, multiple men), polyamorous cultures (multiple people in webs of relationships), "free love" cultures, and entirely abstinent cultures like the Shakers. We've had cultures that shamed homosexual behavior or celebrated it; cultures that shamed women or men, and cultures that shamed everyone; cultures with no gender, two genders, or three or four or five genders.

Which is the right one? Which one is the "natural" or "real" way humans should have sex?

Sex educators and sex therapists want to create a world where all humans everywhere have access to healthful and satisfying sex. Our "ideal" sexual world is one in which every person has the right to decide when and how they touch and are touched, where they have autonomy over their own body and are free to feel how they want to feel about their body and sexuality.

That ideal is what I mean when I use the phrase "sex-positive world." It is the radical, all-inclusive belief that *each person's body belongs to that person.*

Let's imagine a world where all sex, genders, bodies, and loves are "normal," as long as they follow this one rule: that each person's body belongs to that person. No judgment of rightness or wrongness, as long as everyone gets to choose when and how they are touched.

Here is your task in this exercise: Imagine a new mental model of an ideal sexual woman living in a world where there was no "ideal" to which she was supposed to conform. Set her free.

Let's give her a name—maybe it's yours: _____

What does this woman look like, and how does she behave outside sexual situations?

How does she initiate sex, if she does?

What does she do and how does she feel during sex?

How does her partner feel about her sexuality?

What would she *never* do or experience?

from the q & a vault

Q: What's the etiquette for going to a sex toy store?

A: We sex educators have a saying: "Don't yuck anybody's yum." That's sex toy store etiquette, too.

The people who work in sex-positive, gender-inclusive sex toy stores make their living matching people with the toy or lube or garment that will bring that individual pleasure. If there is such a place near you, walk in the door and stay neutral as you browse the shelves. If you see something that's not for you, that's fine, but if it weren't for someone, it wouldn't be in the store. Your "yuck" is someone else's "yum," and your "yum" is someone else's "yuck." Be kind: No yucking.

There will be a lingerie section, a lube section, and a variety of toy sections, maybe organized by type—bullet vibrators, slim-line vibrators, heavy-duty "wand" vibrators, penetration-oriented vibrators. There may also be a book section, a bondage gear and sensation play section, a "packer" and dildo section.

Just reading that list might be enough to trigger a yuck response in you. If so, this is a great opportunity to start practicing noticing that response and just letting it move through you and out, without you having to do a thing about it.

If you notice something that surprises you, you might make a curious little "Huh!" noise. If you notice something that appeals to you, pick it up and explore.

And if you see something you don't like, just notice that, keep your face neutral, and look at something else. Say to yourself, "That's not for me." It's completely fine that it's not for you; remember, sex positivity is about everyone getting to choose how and when they are touched, and people vary in the ways they want to be touched. Imagine how you would feel if someone picked up the toy you thought looked appealing and said, "Ugh, what sort of gross person likes this?"

Ask for help if you want it. In the sex-positive, inclusive sex toy stores, employees are often highly trained to offer accurate information and nonjudgmental support. Their goal is to help you find the right thing for you, whatever that might be.

what do you see that you like?

A sex-positive context is also, by definition, a body-positive context.

The world is decidedly not body positive. By kindergarten, half of girls are worried about being too fat. That number increases through childhood and adolescence, so that by their teenage years, almost all girls have engaged in some kind of weight-control behavior.

Beyond the other (sometimes very serious, even lethal) health consequences of these efforts to conform to the culturally constructed aspirational beauty ideal, does hating your body activate the sexual accelerator?

Heck no. Viewing your body with criticism and disgust only hits the brake.

But it doesn't have to be this way.

This exercise and those that follow are about creating a context that allows you to turn toward your body with kindness and compassion rather than with self-criticism.

First, look at your own naked body in a full-length mirror and write down everything you see *that you like.*

Of course the first thing that will happen is your mind will fill with thoughts about all the parts of yourself you've been told are wrong or bad or disgusting. That's fine; just set those thoughts aside for a few minutes. Look at your body and write down what you like about what you see.

Then do it again the next day.

Do it every day for a week.

Day 1

Day 2

Day 3

Day 4

Day 5

Day 6

Day 7

After seven days of writing down what you see that you like about your body, consider what the experience was like and what changed, if anything.

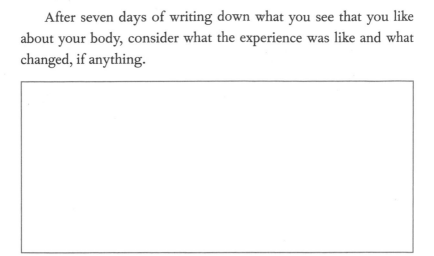

It may feel dissonant at first. It may stay dissonant. That's okay. The goal isn't to eliminate decades of body-based shame and judgment; it's to recognize the pattern of shame and judgment and start asking ourselves if we want to hold on to it or let it go to create space for something else.

This is another exercise that might feel different for trans and nonbinary folks. One reader told me of their first experience shopping for "boy clothes" after a lifetime of shopping in the "girls" and "women's" sections. They said, "I looked at the mannequin (all pectorals and biceps) and had the sinking realization that I now have to look at two body ideals I can never live up to."

It takes an entire lifetime to build up the reflexively self-critical relationship many of us have, where we contrast our bodies with a culturally constructed aspirational ideal. So it will certainly take more than a week to change that relationship to one of compassion and affection. Keep returning to this exercise over time, if you like, and notice how things change.

"she is so beautiful"

You can do this exercise during the same week as exercise 4, or you can do it separately. Instead of looking at your own body, your task in this activity is to notice other people's bodies.

Look at them on the street and on TV, on social media, and as you look, say to yourself, "She is so beautiful."

Intentionally seek out a range of bodies—for example, find the YouTube channel "StyleLikeU," or check out Jes Baker's list of 135 Instagram accounts to diversify your feed.

Just as you might notice your internal yuck response to some sex toys, lubes, or garments, notice your yuck response to some sizes or shapes of bodies. Notice it neutrally, take a breath, and then say to yourself instead, "She is so beautiful."

Because she actually is. "Beautiful" is not something bodies should be, nor is it something they could be if only they conformed with the fantasy ideal. Beautiful is what bodies already are.

Each day, spend a few minutes writing about what it feels like to look for beauty in bodies that don't conform with aspirational beauty ideals.

Day 1

Day 2

Day 3

Day 4

Day 5

Day 6

Day 7

letter to a younger you

Your task with this final activity is to write a letter to a younger version of yourself. Choose an age at which you felt vulnerable about your body: maybe when you were a teenager, maybe just after you had a baby, maybe when you reached menopause. Write a letter to that younger you, telling her what she needed to know about how beautiful she already was and how she could let go of some of the body self-criticism and embrace her body as it was and as it would develop through her life.

one important thing

Take a moment to look back at the exercises in this chapter. Write down one important thing you learned, whether it's about sex in general or about your sexuality in particular:

part three

sex in action

six

arousal

With the deeper understanding you've gained of your body, your brain, and the ways they are shaped by the context in which they develop, it's time to talk about what happens when you actually have sex—and especially what happens when sex doesn't seem to go the way you expect it to. Both this chapter and the next— "Arousal" and "Desire"—are intended to uproot some old and dangerous myths about how sexual response works.

It starts with your brain.

The brain has a mechanism you may have heard called "the reward center," which is composed of three intertwined but separable systems.

First, there's the *liking* system, made up of discrete opioid hot spots in the emotional brain. It assesses the hedonic impact of a stimulus: Does this feel good? How good? Does that feel bad? How bad? Drop sugar water on the tongue of a newborn, and their *liking* system sets off fireworks.

Second, *wanting* is governed by a wide-reaching dopaminergic network in and beyond the emotional brain. It motivates us to move toward or away from a stimulus. It's like your toddler following you around asking for another cookie.

The systems are related, obviously, but they are not identical.

Third and finally, *learning* is a reaction motivated by expectation. Think of how you can ring a bell to train a dog its food is ready. He starts to salivate as soon as the bell rings, before he has even seen the food. Does that mean the dog wants the bell? Or that he thinks the bell is delicious? No. It means the dog has learned that the bell is a food-related stimulus.

When we recognize the separateness of the three systems, we begin to understand a phenomenon researchers call "arousal nonconcordance." That is the topic of this chapter.

Nonconcordance is when a person's physiological response doesn't predict the person's subjective experience.

It happens in every emotional and motivational system. For example, in a study of the "chills" we feel when we hear moving music, some research participants were played "My Heart Will Go On." Half of them reported experiencing chills (subjective experience), and 14 percent exhibited piloerection, where their hair stood on end (physiological response). Other research participants listened to "Bitter Sweet Symphony," by The Verve; 60 percent of them reported chills (subjective experience) and none exhibited piloerection (physiological response).

If their hair stood on end but they did not experience chills, did they get chills? No. And if they said, "I got chills!" but their hair stayed flat, did they get chills? Sure they did. If you're on stage singing and your audience gets chills, who cares what their hair is doing?

Arousal nonconcordance happens with sex, too. Research over

the last thirty years has found that genital blood flow can be activated by cues that are *sex-related*, even if they're not wanted or liked. The overlap between sex-related genital blood flow and liking/wanting subjective arousal ranges between 10 and 50 percent, depending on a variety of factors.

That wide range of overlap means two things. First, people *vary* tremendously—no surprise there. Same parts, organized different ways.

Second, you cannot predict from an individual's genital response to a sex-related stimulus whether they want or like that sex-related stimulus.

pleasure versus arousal

"Pleasure," "desire," and "arousal" are so tangled together in our usual ways of thinking that it takes practice to separate them. In this exercise, spend a few minutes considering your experiences of pleasure and arousal in different contexts.

Step 1. "What does *sexual pleasure* feel like to me?"
How do you know you *like* a sensation? How does it affect your body? Your emotions? Your thoughts?

From your worksheets in chapter 3, reiterate what contexts allow your brain to interpret a sensation as pleasurable:

Contexts that facilitate pleasure	Contexts that don't facilitate pleasure

Step 2. "What does *genital response* feel like to me?"

Some people spontaneously notice their own genital response, and others have to choose to turn their attention to their genitals. When you notice your own genital response, what does it feel like?

From your worksheets in chapter 3, reiterate what contexts allow your brain to interpret genital response as pleasurable:

Contexts where genital response feels good	Contexts where genital response doesn't feel good

Step 3. Take a look at your "How Did You Learn?" exercise back in chapter 2 and your great and not-so-great sexual experiences explored in chapter 3. Did you or a partner experience arousal nonconcordance in any of those instances?

Rewrite the narrative of that experience, keeping the ideas of genital response, pleasure, and desire distinct. What were the sex-related stimuli? What did you like, and what didn't you like? What did you want? How did your partner, if any, respond in that situation?

Every time you use a word to express pleasure, desire, or genital response, mark those words differently, to make sure you're keeping those ideas distinct.

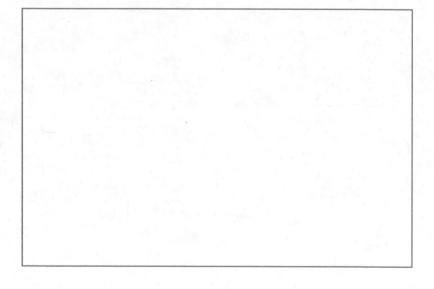

Why does arousal nonconcordance happen? We don't know yet. But, from a day-to-day-life point of view, it doesn't matter.

It is a fascinating scientific question, why bodies respond sometimes and not others. It will be really cool to watch researchers untangle the context-sensitive responses of bodies to sex-related stimuli and how those responses relate to subjective pleasure and desire. But we do not have to wait for the science to advance before we know what's true:

Bodies don't say yes or no;
they say sex-related or not sex-related.

And we live in a sufficiently screwed-up world where some things that are related to sex are neither wanted nor liked, so sometimes our genitals respond when the rest of us isn't interested, and sometimes our genitals don't respond when the rest of us is ready to go.

A student sent me a note after I gave a lecture about arousal nonconcordance. (Warning, this is a story about sexual violence.)

She was with a new partner, doing things she was mostly comfortable with, and when they reached a point where she didn't want to go further, she said no.

Her partner said, "You're wet; you're so ready. Don't be shy."

Shy, as if it hadn't taken all her confidence and courage to say no to someone she liked, whose feelings she didn't want to hurt.

She said it again. "No."

Did he listen to her words?

No.

She never told anyone what happened until she wrote to me; because her body responded, she thought she couldn't call it rape.

Sometimes consent is ambiguous. But let's make sure we're noticing how clear consent often is, once we eliminate this myth.

"But you were wet," or "Well, you got an erection, so . . ." These are used to discredit survivors of sexual violence. Survivors know they didn't want it or like it and still sometimes their bodies respond—and this goes for all survivors, no matter their genitals or gender identity or sexual orientation. People who experience genital response during sexual assault sometimes describe feeling betrayed by their bodies, because they were taught this myth that genital response implies liking or wanting.

Understanding arousal nonconcordance doesn't just improve your own sex life, though it can definitely do that. It helps you support and believe survivors (and that might include yourself) whose bodies didn't respond the way they were taught to expect.

noticing when people mistake arousal for pleasure or desire

Now that you know about arousal nonconcordance, you'll notice every time people get it wrong. Journalists get it wrong, when they're reporting on the arousal nonconcordance research, like this example from a feminist, sex-positive writer:

> When [researcher Meredith] Chivers showed a group of women a procession of videos of naked women, naked men, heterosexual sex, gay sex, lesbian sex, and bonobo sex, her subjects "were turned on right away by all of it, including the copulating apes." But when it came time to self-report their arousal, the survey and the plethysmograph [a device that measures genital blood flow] "hardly matched at all," [writer Daniel] Bergner reports. Straight women claimed to respond to straight sex more than they really did; lesbian women claimed to respond to straight sex far less than they really did; nobody admitted a response to the bonobo sex. Physically, female desire seemed "omnivorous," but mentally, it revealed "an objective and subjective divide."

Circle or highlight the words that show she's mistaking arousal for pleasure or desire.

Imagine a friend sends you this article to read. What would you say to the friend, to clarify the distinctions among arousal, pleasure, and desire?

And here's philosopher Alain de Botton, in *How to Think More About Sex*:

> Erections and lubrication simply cannot be effected by will-power and are therefore particularly true and honest indices of interest. In a world in which fake enthusiasms are rife, in which it is often hard to tell whether people really like us or whether they are being kind to us merely out of a sense of duty, the wet vagina and the stiff penis function as unambiguous agents of sincerity.

Circle or highlight the words that show he's mistaking arousal for pleasure or desire. What would you say to this author, to clarify the distinctions among arousal, pleasure, and desire?

The more you practice noticing this mistake and describing how arousal is not pleasure or desire, desire is not arousal or pleasure, and pleasure is not arousal or desire, the better you'll be able to talk to your partners about all these aspects of sexuality, and the more readily you'll be able to spot when a message in the media is reinforcing the myth that genitals know more about what a person wants or likes than the person does.

from the q & a vault

Q: **Can you suggest a healthy lube?**

A: Can I ever!

Even when your genital response matches your arousal level, our natural fluids are rarely adequate to prevent chafing, tearing, and pain that come with the friction of body parts rubbing together. So anyone who has sex that involves genital contact should try using a lubricant—especially if there's penetration involved. Lube will reduce friction, which not only reduces pain and increases pleasure, but also reduces tearing, which reduces the risk of sexually transmitted infection. Lube is as much about health as it is about pleasure.

Everyone's body and personal preferences are different, and there's usually more than one good lube to choose from. Here's a handful of great resources to help you find what's right for you:

- Tool Shed, a sex toy store in Milwaukee, Wisconsin, has a "Lube 101" section on its website, which makes an excellent place to start.
- Good Vibrations, for those who prefer spreadsheets over unstructured browsing, offers a comprehensive "lube chart" organized by main ingredient.
- The website for Smitten Kitten, a sex toy store in Minneapolis, Minnesota, is a hub for science-loving readers with their comprehensive guide to lube, including the pH levels of many lubes and an explanation of how osmolality (!) influences the quality of a lube.

say the words

Practice communicating clearly about the distinction between what you want, what you like, and what causes genital blood flow. Practice saying the words. Some examples:

- "Genital response just means something is sex-related; it doesn't mean it's wanted or liked. It's called arousal nonconcordance."
- "Some people think your body doesn't respond when you don't want or like it. If only that were true! Instead, genitals can respond to any sex-related stimulation, even if it grosses the person out."
- "If your mouth watered when you ate some rotten fruit, nobody would ever say, 'You just don't want to *admit* you like it.' Same goes for genitals."
- "My genitals don't tell you what I want or like. I do."

Imagine your partner says, "But you're so wet!" or "But you're not wet!" when you express a level of pleasure or desire that doesn't match your genital response. What could you say to help them be a great sex partner?

Imagine a friend makes a mean-spirited joke about "She said no, but her body said 'yes." What could you say to help them understand what such a joke gets wrong?

And finally, imagine a friend or partner tells you about a time when they were sexually assaulted, and they mention that their body responded. What could you say to help them understand what their genital response meant?

one important thing

Take a moment to look back at the exercises in this chapter. Write down one important thing you learned, whether it's about sex in general or about your sexuality in particular:

desire

"Desire differential"—that is, one partner wanting sex more than the other—is the most common reason couples seek sex therapy, and loss of desire is women's most commonly reported sexual issue. So it's not surprising that I get asked about desire more than anything else, most often in a question like, "Emily, how do couples sustain a strong sexual connection over the long term?"

This chapter answers that question.

what to expect from desire

How does desire work, how does it change, and what's "normal"?

When we look at the research on couples who sustain a strong sexual connection over multiple decades, we find that these are not couples who constantly crave sex. Nor are they couples who have sex often—very few couples have sex more than a couple of times a week; people are busy. Nor do they have wildly adventurous sex. On the contrary, one recent study found that the best predictor of sex and relationship satisfaction wasn't frequency of sex or what a couple did or even whether they had orgasms. The best predictor of sex and relationship satisfaction was whether they cuddled after sex.

Generally, the couples who sustain a strong sexual connection over the long term seem to have two things in common:

One: They are friends—even best friends. Their relationship has, at its core, a deep trust. Therapist and relationship researcher Sue Johnson boils trust down to this question: "Are you there for me?" Friends are there for each other.

Two: They prioritize sex. They decide that it matters for their relationship that they set aside the mundane aspects of their shared life—jobs, kids, friends, sleep, or even, god forbid, just some television. They close the door on all those things, and they show up. They put their bodies in the bed. They let their skin touch their partner's skin, and their body remembers, *Oh right, I like this. I like this person.*

That's it! Best friends. Prioritize sex.

This is not the story we usually hear about how sexual desire works. In some ways, it contradicts everything about the mainstream idea of sexual desire. Check out your "ideal" women in chapter 5. Did any of them have "prioritize sex with her best friend" as their "perfect sex"?

The narrative many of us learn is "spontaneous desire." Erika Moen, the cartoonist who illustrated *Come As You Are*, draws spontaneous desire as a lightning bolt to the genitals—ka-*boom!* It seems to appear out of the blue, in anticipation of pleasure.

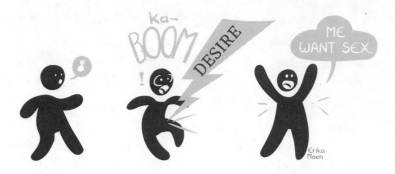

Spontaneous desire can be fun, and it's certainly one normal, healthy way to experience sexual desire, but there's another desire style called "responsive desire." Where spontaneous desire emerges apparently in *anticipation* of pleasure, responsive desire emerges in *response* to pleasure.

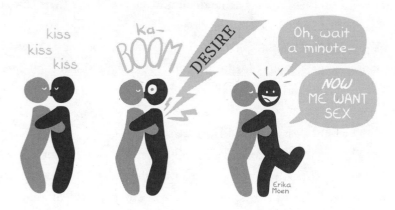

Another way to put it:

Pleasure is the measure.

Pleasure is the measure of sexual wellbeing. It's not how much you ka-*boom!* crave sex, it's not how often you do it, what you do, or where, or how many orgasms you have. It's whether or not you *like the sex you are having.* After all, why would you desire sex if the sex isn't pleasurable?

If you're struggling to differentiate spontaneous and responsive desire, consider this analogy from sex therapist Christine Hyde:

If your best friend invites you to a party, of course you accept, because it's your best friend and a party! But maybe as the date approaches you start to worry about arranging child care or dreading the traffic, and when the night arrives you don't feel like putting on your party clothes after a long day at work. But you said you would go, so you put on your party clothes and you go. And what happens? Usually you have fun at the party! If you're having fun, you're doing it right.

That's responsive desire.

Spontaneous desire in this analogy would be the sudden urge to go to a party, even if there was no party planned.

And consider this: if you had been to this friend's parties a dozen times and they were always duds, with food you didn't enjoy and people you didn't quite trust, would any amount of *wanting* to go to a party make that party worth going to?

contexts that create desire

Some people experience exclusively spontaneous desire, and others experience exclusively responsive desire, but most people experience both, at different times in their lives.

Why? Because desire, like pleasure, is shaped by context.

In this exercise, you'll think through some experiences of spontaneous and responsive desire and consider what aspects of the context facilitated those experiences of desire.

This exercise will feel familiar. In exercises 1 and 2 in chapter 3—"Consider the Context" and "Assess the Context"—you explored how the context shaped your experience of *pleasure*. Here you'll consider how the context shapes your experience of *desire*. In exercise 2 in chapter 2—"What Turns On the Ons, What Turns Off the Offs?"—you noticed the factors that reliably shut off all desire or some that reliably activate desire, regardless of what other contextual factors may be at play.

Now when you consider the great and not-so-great sexual experiences you've had, what contextual factors seem to facilitate positive experiences of responsive desire? Which facilitate positive experiences of spontaneous desire?

Contexts That Shut Off Desire	Contexts That Facilitate Responsive Desire	Contexts That Facilitate Spontaneous Desire

As always, you may decide to work toward creating contexts that facilitate either experience of desire. Go back to the "creating change" worksheets to think through a plan.

what do you want when you want sex?

This exercise is for a partner who wants more sex than their partner does.

You know from experience that spontaneous desire can be pleasurable in some contexts, but it can also be uncomfortable in other contexts. In what contexts is desire *not* pleasurable?

Contexts When Spontaneous Desire Is Pleasurable	Contexts When Spontaneous Desire Is Not Pleasurable

Now here is the most important part. Given everything you know about the contexts that facilitate spontaneous desire and which of those contexts make spontaneous desire feel good or not-so-good, ask yourself this:

"What do I want when I want sex?"

The answer isn't just orgasm—you can have an orgasm on your own. What is it about sex with this person that feels so important?

Some questions to help you brainstorm:

- When your partner declines your invitation to sex, what does your body or heart feel is being rejected, apart from sex itself?
- When they accept, what does it feel like they are accepting?
- If your partner rarely or never initiates, what does that seem to mean to you?
- If your partner has responsive desire, is there part of you that judges their desire style as "less normal" than your spontaneous desire; that wishes they had spontaneous desire; or imagines that if they loved you enough or found you sexy enough, they'd have spontaneous desire? Responsive desire has nothing to do with how much they love you or how attractive they find you, but does it feel that way?

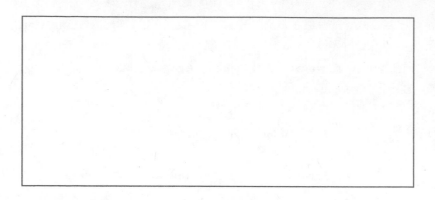

Telling your partner what you really want when you want sex won't necessarily make them agree to have sex with you more often, but it will open up clearer channels of communication and even create ways for you to get those needs met nonsexually! And when you're feeling like your needs are met, you will feel less compelled to "chase" after sex from your partner, which will relieve their sense of obligation (and sometimes failure and resentment), which will release their brake a bit, and may even ultimately lead to better sex.

Q: **I love my partner, but don't feel that physical passion and connection. How can I get that back?**

A: You put your body in the bed, you let your skin touch your partner's skin, and you allow yourself to remember how much you like this person, how much you enjoy sex. Remember: pleasure is the measure, not how much "passion" you feel for your partner or how much you spontaneously desire them or they desire you, but how much pleasure you experience when you connect sexually. Remove the things that are hitting your brakes and allow the accelerator to be activated.

Connection is created by connecting. If you feel a lack of connection, then connect, whether erotically, emotionally, or intellectually.

There is an exception: if the problem is not merely lack of connection, but active dread, seek outside help.

To illustrate: A few years ago, I was sitting in a bar with a couple of friends over some beers. Married couple, seven academic degrees and two young children between them. Big nerds, very in love, but very sleep deprived. They asked the question I get asked most often: How could they sustain a strong sexual connection over the long term? I told them about responsive desire and about best friends prioritizing sex. I said, "The ludic factor means you put your body in the bed and let your skin touch your partner's skin and—"

As I said that, one of the partners literally cringed away from the table.

It wasn't just that she didn't want sex; she *dreaded* sex.

It happens all the time. Nice people who love each other come to dread sex. Sometimes a sex therapist seeing such a couple will ask them to stand up and face each other, then create as much physical space between them as they need to feel comfortable, and the less-interested partner might create twenty feet of space.

And that space is not empty. It's crowded with accumulated hurt and resentment blocking the partners: *you're not listening* and *if you loved me* and *I don't know what's wrong with me but your criticism isn't helping* and *you're not there for me*—years, maybe, of hurt feelings, forming a blockage between partners. These are the cause of the dread.

This happens in any relationship that lasts long enough; you, too, are fostering a blockage of hurt feelings with your certain special someone. The couples who sustain strong sexual connections are not the ones with no blockages—they're the ones who know how to clear it out. Which is to say, they are not couples who never hurt each other; they're the ones who find their way back.

Does the blockage between you and your partner appear overwhelming to you? Consider finding a sex therapist to help you sort through the issues creating the blockage.

transitioning into "the mood"

This exercise is for people whose experience of desire is primarily responsive.

Responsive folks often need to *plan* sex, just as you plan a party. You put it in your calendar—as in Saturday at 3 p.m., you, your certain special someone, and the red underwear—and you show up when you said you would.

People sometimes ask me, "If you have to plan it, doesn't that mean you don't want it enough?"

On the contrary. Is there anything we do that really matters to us that we don't plan? If something is important to us, if we want it enough, we make time for it in our busy lives and our packed schedules. Sex must matter a lot if you're willing to block out time on your calendar for it.

Your goal with that scheduled time is to create a *protected space* where you connect sexually with your certain special someone. In game design parlance, this protected space is called a "magic circle," where you shift into a different state of mind, one that is ready to focus on pleasure.

Once you embrace the idea of scheduling sex and creating a magic circle—which is what many couples who sustain a long-term sexual connection do—the most difficult step for responsive folks is the deliberate transition from their day-to-day state of mind into a magic-circle state of mind. How do you get from "I just have too many other things I need to take care of and worry about and finish!" to "All my attention is focused on pleasure and my partner and our shared connection."

To figure out how to transition from everyday life into the

magic circle, let's return to the skills we practiced in exercise 4, "Planning for Change," in chapter 3.

1. **Planful problem-solving.** Say to yourself, "If I decided to transition from my everyday state of mind to a magic-circle state of mind, here's what would go on my to-do list."
2. **Reverse engineering.** Imagine what it will be like after you've made the transition, and then think backward. What did you do to get there?
3. **Strengths-based.** You've found your way to the magic circle before. What strengths do you possess that allowed you to make the transition?

To transition into a magic-circle state of mind, I . . .

Common transition activities include completing the stress response cycle (see chapter 4); reinforcing the sense of connection with your partner by talking about how you met, what you admire about each other, or great sex you've had before; doing explicitly erotic things, whether with your partner or alone—e.g., touching each other's bodies, watching porn you like together, or reading erotica on your own in the bathtub; practicing rituals of safety and welcome, like lighting candles or reciting familiar words; or "getting ready for the party": caring for your body and decorating it in ways that make you feel glorious.

Now let's create a hypothetical plan. In the space below, describe your plan for transitioning into the magic circle, including a hypothetical date when you might schedule an opportunity for sex.

Name of Plan (e.g., "Operation Magic Sexylady"): _____

Start Date: _____

Description of Plan:

What behavioral, emotional, physical, or interpersonal cues will show you your plan is working?

Finally, anticipate the likely barriers that might prevent you from being able to follow through on your plan, and choose a strategy for handling that barrier should it arise.

Likely Barrier	Strategy for Handling It

As usual, you may choose to pursue this plan if it's important enough to you and you feel confident enough (see chapter 3), or you may prefer not to begin yet.

five initiation styles

How do you invite your partner in? How does your partner invite you? How do you *wish* they'd invite you? Each sexual experience has to start somewhere—in other words, someone probably initiates that sex. Different people have different preferences when it comes to initiation. Sex therapist Petra Zebroff's Sexual Initiation Scale of Arousal identifies five general initiation styles:

1. *The Provocative Seduction Style:* It is the "game of seduction" that gets them to feel that erotic connection. They want to see your desire for them—with a little skin, signs of arousal, undressing or posing for their delight. Being approached with provocative teasing, playful hints, or words of desire ("I want you. I need you right now") helps them feel erotic.

2. *The Sensual Touch Style:* From caressing their neck to massage to direct genital contact—physical touch is what creates a context that opens them up to erotic connection.

3. *The Emotional Connection Style:* Responds to sweetness, romantic gestures, and connecting conversation. Demonstrations of love and sharing are central to moving them into the erotic realm. Being genuinely seen and understood by a partner creates a context that opens them up to erotic connection.

4. *The Sex Talk Style:* Whether it's hearing how sexy they look or being told what their partner wants to do to them, direct sexual words are what create a context that opens them up to erotic connection.

5. *The Power Play Style:* Focused attention and creating a power differential—either being in control or being controlled—are the contexts that open them up to erotic connection. Being approached with *confidence* and *urgency.*

Provocative Seduction	Sensual Touch	Emotional Connection
• Sends me or shows me sexy pics • Takes a provocative pose or shows more skin • Hints or jokes about sex • Engages me in planning a sexual event or scene • Wears or doesn't wear certain articles of clothing • Undresses for me • Tells me directly that they want to have sex	• Caresses all parts of my body including nonsexual parts • Kisses or caresses my neck • Starts slow • Gives me gentle kisses • Touches my back or buttocks • Wakes me up with kisses or sexual touch • Strokes my chest or plays with my nipples • Gives me a massage	• Acts genuinely interested in what I have to say • Arranges quality time, such as a romantic dinner/event • Addresses concerns/worries I might have • Makes me laugh, laughs easily • Engages in an intellectual or romantic conversation • Tells me how much he/she loves me • Does something genuinely caring or thoughtful

Above you'll find a wide range of initiation techniques (how you would want your partner to initiate sex with you), adapted from Petra Zebroff's Sexual Initiation Scale of Arousal, to help you assess your own and your partner's initiation styles. Draw a line through any initiation action that doesn't sound appealing to you. Circle the ones that seem like they could be fun in the right context. Add a star to the initiation actions that would be appealing in almost any context.

Sex Talk	Power Play
• Tells me how sexy I am or how much they desire me • Tells me the things he/she wants to do to me • Talks dirty to me • Sends me a sexy message	• Pushes me against a wall or bed • Takes charge of the situation • Is rough or forceful • Demands that they have me immediately • Approaches me from behind • Surprises me or is spontaneous

You may notice that one or two of the styles are most appealing to you, while others are less appealing. This indicates your initiation style—that is, the type of stimulation that's likely to hit your accelerator. As with desire style, most people are a mixture of more than one, depending on the context. And as with arousal, just because it activates the accelerator doesn't necessarily mean it's pleasurable. You can use this exercise to talk with your partner about what works for you each individually and what works for you as partners to each other.

•   •   •

When it comes to sexual pleasure, you don't have to wait for "the mood."

Waiting to be in the mood too often means waiting for your life to be calm enough for you not to be stressed, and because many of us sustain a state of stress for years at a time, waiting for the mood means waiting indefinitely. And worse, the more you wait, the more frustration, isolation, and worry builds up between you and your partner. "Am I broken? Are they? Is our relationship doomed?"

The mood comes when there's enough stimulation on the accelerator and enough turning off of the brakes. A great way to help your partner's brakes turn off is to make sure they feel attractive, supported, admired, and—this is crucial—under no obligation to want sex!

one important thing

Take a moment to look back at the exercises in this chapter. Write down one important thing you learned, whether it's about sex in general or about your sexuality in particular:

part four

ecstasy for everybody

eight

orgasm

People have a lot of feelings about orgasm. We wish we could have more of them, more easily, or through different kinds of stimulation. And much of the distress and longing people experience is based not on any problem with orgasm, but on a misleading cultural script about what orgasms are and how they work.

So let's start simply, with a definition.

> Orgasm is the sudden, involuntary release of tension
> generated in response to sex-related stimuli.

Notice how much is missing from that definition: there's no mention of genitals, muscle contractions, any specific sexual behavior, pleasure, or indeed anything that specifies what it feels like or how it happened. Orgasms *vary*—from woman to woman and from context to context. They happen while you're making love—and sometimes they don't. They happen while you're masturbating—and sometimes they don't. They can happen from clitoral stimulation, vaginal stimulation, thigh stimulation, anal stimulation, breast stimulation, earlobe stimulation, or from mental stimulation with no physical contact at all—or not during any of these. They can happen while you're asleep, while you're exercising, or while you're in a variety of other completely nonsexual situations. They can be delightful, humdrum, spiritual, annoying, ecstatic, fun, or frustrating. Sometimes they're great. Sometimes they're not. Sometimes you want them. Sometimes you don't.

All orgasms are different, and there is no "better" kind of orgasm. It's even hard to say that there are "different kinds" of orgasm—except that they're all made of the same basic processes (sudden, involuntary release of sexual tension) organized in different ways, and there are different ways to make them happen.

Despite the efforts of women's magazines (and even scientists) to identify and label the various kinds of orgasms we could be having—G-spot orgasms, blended orgasms, uterine orgasms, vulval orgasms, and all the rest—what it comes down to is a sudden, involuntary release of sexual tension, generated in different ways.

It's true that orgasms generated through different kinds of stimulation often *feel* different. But it's also true that different orgasms on different days, stimulated the same way, feel different from each other, because the context is different. We know by now that context shapes whether and how intensely a sensation feels pleasurable. And all orgasms are normal and healthy, regardless of what kind of stimulation generated them or how they feel. Their "quality" comes not from how it came to be or whether or not it meets some arbitrary criteria, but from whether or not you liked it and wanted it.

Distress about orgasm is the second most common reason people seek treatment for sexual problems (after desire). It occurs in about 5 to 15 percent of women overall, though a quarter of American women in their twenties have yet to experience orgasm, as far as they know. And there probably are some women who never experience orgasm, though it's not clear how many of them are not able to orgasm under *any* circumstances, and how many are just not interested enough to keep looking for the right context. I met a woman in Boston who had had her first orgasm in her seventies, so I'm inclined to believe that any woman interested enough in sex to want to have an orgasm *can* have an orgasm.

This chapter is for those who want to get to know their orgasms more intimately, or even meet their orgasm for the first time.

from the q & a vault

Q: How do I know if I've ever had an orgasm?

A: Orgasm is like being tickled or spanked or caressed or hugged: how a sensation feels depends on the context. Sometimes it can be fun, other times it's annoying, and sometimes it feels like almost nothing. Pleasure is a perception of a sensation, and perception is context dependent. That's just as true for orgasm as it is for tickling or spanking. So it's not too surprising that a person might have difficulty distinguishing orgasm from other kinds of sexual pleasure.

The basic principle is: Do you feel like you had an orgasm? Then you did. Rhythmic contractions of the pelvic floor muscle are the most typical sensation associated with orgasm, but it's not universal. In general, orgasm (which is the sudden, involuntary release of sexual tension) will feel like you're spontaneously "done" in some way. A lot of people feel "finished." Others feel like they're ready to get going. Some people's genitals may feel numb and unresponsive; others' may feel so ultrasensitive that any touch is irritating.

But overall, orgasms are like art: you know it when you see it.

normalizing masturbation

The vast majority of women masturbate, and rates of masturbation have been going up for as long as science has been asking. In the 1953 Kinsey Report on women's sexual behavior, 62 percent of the women interviewed reported having masturbated at least once in their lives. By 1973, 82 percent of women interviewed for the Hite Report said they had masturbated at least once. And by 2013, when researchers asked again, 91 percent of women reported that they had masturbated at least once. About half of women—between 30 and 70 percent, depending on age—have masturbated in the last year.

This also means nearly 10 percent of women don't masturbate, and that's normal, too. If you don't want to masturbate, that's totally fine, and the exercises in this chapter can be adapted for use with a partner very easily, or practiced without genital touching.

But if you do masturbate or you're willing to try masturbation, you can set aside any thought that it is anything other than a normal, common, healthy way to experience sexual stimulation.

For our purposes, "masturbation" means sexually stimulating yourself when you're alone. It is arguably the most stigmatized sexual behavior of all, yet it is the most efficient—and the most commonly suggested by sex therapists—way to explore your own experience of orgasm. Getting okay with the idea of touching your own body is an important first step toward exploring orgasm and all the ways you might experience it. To that end, let's take a look at how much women vary in their masturbation technique.

There is no "right" or "wrong" way to masturbate, and if you don't generally masturbate, that's fine, too. Many modes of masturbation have been catalogued by various researchers across the decades, including:

Postures: lying on your back, lying on your stomach, lying on your side, standing up, and holding the pelvis still or rocking the pelvis in any of these postures

Technique: hand, vibrator, water massage, pressing your thighs together rhythmically, rubbing your pelvis against an object (e.g., furniture or a pillow)

On the chart below, indicate: (1) which modes of masturbation you used during your earliest experiences of masturbation; (2) which modes of masturbation you used when you last masturbated; (3) which modes of masturbation are most typical for you; (4) which modes of masturbation you have rarely or never used but might be interested in trying.

	Hand	Vibrator or other object	Water massage	Pressing thighs together	Rubbing against an object (e.g., furniture or a pillow)
On your back					
On your stomach					
On your side					
Standing up					
Other:					

Take a moment to notice what it feels like to think in this systematic way about your masturbation technique. Was there a difference between this exercise and the previous exercises? Did some part of you hesitate to mark this page in case anyone saw it? What would happen if they did?

Other modes of stimulation to consider:

Do you penetrate your vagina? Regardless of what you may have learned from porn, the vast majority of women masturbate *without* vaginal penetration most of the time, focusing instead on the labia and clitoris. Penetrating the vagina during masturbation is normal, too! But don't trust what you may have seen in porn as a representation of the only "right" way to touch your body for your own pleasure.

Do you keep your pelvis still ("pelvic-passive") when you masturbate, or do you rock your pelvis ("pelvic-active")? Perhaps your pelvis is active during some kinds of stimulation and still during others—or perhaps it's the same regardless of stimulation.

	Pelvic-active	Pelvic-passive
Mostly external stimulation		
Definitely some internal stimulation		

The exercises that follow will ask you to touch your own body—sometimes sexually, and sometimes not. How you prefer to touch yourself is up to you, and you have 100 percent permission to try new things and touch your body in whatever way you're interested in exploring.

noticing sensations and your feelings about those sensations

Because the plan in this chapter is to expand sexual pleasure, the first step is noticing general sensations and your feelings about those sensations. Most of us have been taught to shut out signals from at least some of our body parts, so learning to tune in will reconnect you with sensation. Your task with this exercise is to notice what various sensations feel like in your body and to notice how you instinctively react to those sensations, while you pay neutral, nonjudgmental attention to your complete internal experience.

(For those who don't struggle with orgasm, this exercise may appear too "beginner," so you might be inclined to skip it. Try it anyway. You'll be surprised at how it can take you from someone who doesn't struggle with orgasm to someone who has explosive, mind-bending orgasms.)

Step 1. Using what you've learned in chapters 2 through 5, describe a context or two where your brain and body have access to pleasure. It doesn't have to be orgasmic or ecstatic pleasure, but plain, simple enjoyment of sensations, including touch, on your own. For most people, this will be a time when you don't feel rushed or fear interruption. What context could you create for yourself where you would feel free to explore the sensations of your body?

Step 2. Choose a day and time when you can create that context, and get yourself into a space where you feel good. Take off your clothes and get comfortable. Then do some nongenital touching. Touch all of your body *except your genitals* in whatever way feels interesting to you. Play with all the different sensations your nervous system can sense, in all the different places it can sense them.

Types of sensations include light touch, like a caress; deep touch, like massage; temperature; vibration; pain, both light (pinprick) and deep (muscle ache); proprioception (the position of your limbs and body in space); interoception (the sensations of your internal processes, such as digestion); and stretching of muscles and connective tissue. Play with sensations. Explore. Sensations may change if you sustain them for a while—for example, holding a stretch or keeping your hand still versus continuously moving it. The effects of sensation may continue past the touch, such as the ongoing sting after you smack an area or the gradual relaxation after you tense a muscle.

Some body parts to touch include your hair and scalp; your ears, face, jaw, neck, and throat; your shoulders and back; your upper arms; elbows (inside and outside) and forearms; your waist and belly; your hips and buttocks; your thighs; your knees (inside and out); your calves; and your feet—the tops and soles, arches and heels, and each of your toes, both left and right. Not everyone has all these parts, not everyone likes the parts they have, and not everyone can reach all their parts. That's okay. You don't have to use your hands—you can touch one foot with your other foot, or touch your foot against your knee, noticing both the sensation of your knee and the sensation of your foot. Rub your legs against each other, rub your arms against your torso.

Some responses to notice:

Guarding: Physicians being trained to diagnose pain are taught that patients may "guard" against pain, bracing themselves with tension in anticipation of contact they expect will hurt. Are there areas of your body or kinds of sensation/touch that made your body want to guard or protect itself, moving away from the touch?

Self-criticism: As we explored in chapter 5, many of us are taught to be dissatisfied with parts of our bodies because they don't match the cultural aspirational ideal. Are there parts of your body that activate self-critical thoughts and feelings? What does that criticism feel like to those parts? What happens if you try turning toward those parts with gratitude, kindness, and compassion for all the times they've tolerated that criticism?

Disgust: In chapter 5 we also talked about "yuck" responses. Is there any body part that triggers a sense of disgust or avoidance in you? What is it like to live in a body 24/7 when parts of that body disgust you? Ask that part how it feels about your disgust, and listen compassionately to its answer. What happens if you try experiencing those parts as neutral?

Safety: Is there a particular body part or type of sensation that activates a sense of safety inside your body? How do you experience safety in your body, thoughts, and emotions?

Practice this multiple times, whether every day for a week or once a week for seven weeks. Write down what the experiences are like for you:

Day 1

Day 2

Day 3

Day 4

Day 5

Day 6

Day 7

172

replace frustration with curiosity

The most common word women use to describe their struggle with orgasm is "frustrated."

Frustration hits the brake, and most problems with orgasm are due to too many things hitting the brakes, so let's reduce frustration.

The opposite of frustration is *curiosity*.

To facilitate curiosity, change your goal: stop trying to have an orgasm. Orgasm is off the table for now.

Instead of orgasm, *exploration* is the new goal.

Here's how:

Step 1. Create a sex-positive context that can be interruption free for at least fifteen minutes—at *least*. Half an hour would be great.

Step 2. As you did in exercise 2, take off your clothes and get comfortable, then experience some general sensations.

Then allow your attention to move to your genitals.

For a few minutes, don't touch your genitals physically; just focus your attention on that area of your body.

When you're ready, touch your genitals. (Be sure your hands are washed and your fingernails well groomed.) You might want to use some kind of lubricant on your fingers. Start with light touch, then incorporate as many of the types of sensation as you want—pressure, pinching, temperature, stretching, sustained or fleeting, internal and external. Notice what all those sensations feel like. If you become aroused, that's fine. Just notice that. Right now the goal is to notice sensations with curiosity, without doing anything about it.

Notice, too, the ways genital sensations affect other parts of your body. Do you experience muscle tension? Does your breathing change? Are there sensations in your face or legs or feet? Be curious about the sensations.

And notice all the responses to sensations from the previous exercise—guarding, self-criticism, disgust, and safety. Be curious about those, too.

Explore the sensations of your genitals for five to ten minutes before you transition back to nongenital touch and then back to the external world. Write what the experience is like for you.

practicing ecstasy

The most important "turn off the offs" practice of all is self-kindness. Too often I've seen women get stuck in their sexual growth because they can't get past their belief that something "shouldn't" hit their brakes. It "shouldn't" turn them off to have the lights on, they "shouldn't" be so hung up about their bodies.

Does believing your sexuality "should" be different from what it is activate the accelerator?

Nope. Brakes.

That's why sex educators have a saying: stop "shoulding" on yourself.

If you wanted to, how would you stop shoulding on yourself and instead begin to embrace your body's full capacity for ecstatic pleasure?

Practice and a sex-positive context.

You already know how to create a sex-positive context—the worksheets from chapters 3, 4, and 7 help you with that.

Which leaves us with the practice part.

Your task in this exercise is to explore with curiosity a wide range of intensities of sexual pleasure.

Begin as you did in exercise 3, with general sensations, then allow your thoughts and touch to go to erotic places. This time, let your arousal grow. Imagine the landscape of your sexual pleasure and response on a scale from zero (a neutral state with no sexual pleasure or response) to ten (ecstasy). Allow yourself to get to a four.

Then stop and let your arousal level diminish back to a one.

This is what I call an "arousal cycle."

Pause and take a moment to write down any thoughts, emotions, or physical sensations this process of arousal and de-arousal may have brought up.

You can stop the exercise here if you like, or you can keep going.

If you choose to go on, let your arousal grow up to five. And back to one. This is your second arousal cycle.

Pause again, and take a moment to write down any thoughts, emotions, or physical sensations you may have noticed.

Again, you can stop the exercise here, or you may choose to keep going. This time, let your arousal process go up to six. And down to two. This is your third arousal cycle.

Pause and take a moment to write down any thoughts, emotions, or physical sensations.

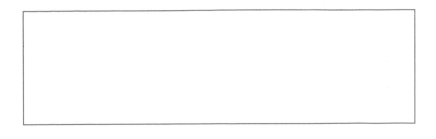

You can continue this way more or less indefinitely—letting your arousal grow to an eight, then down to a three, then an eight and a half, down to a four, then to a nine and down to a five. Then up to a nine and a half, on the teetering edge of orgasm, then down to a six.

And so on, approaching and then backing away from increasingly intense sexual pleasure. The higher the intensity of the arousal, the more gradually you should approach it, so that you never cross over that edge into orgasm.

Your goal is to notice the sensations with curiosity. You're not trying to have an orgasm; you're just exploring the various ways you experience sexual pleasure throughout your body, at different levels of intensity.

If you notice your body wanting to move toward orgasm, just notice that and back away. Take a deep breath. Relax your abdomen. Remind yourself that orgasm is not the goal, pleasure is the goal. Are you experiencing pleasure? Then you're doing it right, exploring your sexual landscape with curiosity. You can conclude this exercise in whatever way feels right for you. You might want to let yourself orgasm, if not having one will leave you feeling frustrated, or you might not. You might prefer to allow that sexual tension to stay in your body and see what that feels like.

Try it every day for a week, or one day a week for seven weeks, allowing your body to access higher intensities of arousal each time. Be sure to note each arousal cycle you experience, each day.

Day 1

Day 2

Day 3

Day 4

Day 5

Day 6

Day 7

You were born entitled to all the pleasure your body can feel, in whatever way your body experiences it, in whatever contexts create it, and in whatever quantities you want it. Your pleasure belongs to you, to share or keep as you choose, to explore or not as you choose, to embrace or avoid as you choose.

one important thing

Take a moment to look back at the exercises in this chapter. Write down one important thing you learned, whether it's about sex in general or about your sexuality in particular:

nine

a new script

We've learned about a lot of brain mechanisms so far—the dual control model, context sensitivity, the liking/wanting/learning system. Here's one more:

In your brain, there is a little "monitor" who observes you as you work toward a goal. She knows (a) what your goal is, (b) how much effort you're investing, and (c) how much progress you're making. So she is aware of the ratio of effort to progress.

She has a very strong opinion about what that ratio should be.

You experience that opinion as an "expectancy," and it profoundly influences your state of mind. When the monitor feels that you're making good progress, you feel great—motivated, eager. But when the monitor feels that you're not making enough progress toward your goal, relative to the effort you're investing, she grows *frustrated*, which motivates you to increase your effort to make more progress toward the goal.

If you still aren't making enough progress to satisfy the little monitor, she gets angry, and then enraged! And eventually, if you continue to fall short, at a certain point the monitor gives up and pushes you off an emotional cliff into a pit of despair, as the monitor becomes convinced that the goal is unattainable. You give up in hopeless despair.

When you're continually failing to reach a sexual goal, whether it's orgasm or spontaneous desire or hearing your partner say yes to sex, your little monitor makes you frustrated, then angry, then eventually despairing.

Do you suppose frustration, anger, or despair hit the accelerator, or do they hit the brake?

How you feel about your sexuality is a major influence on your sexual wellbeing, and this monitor mechanism is the key to shaping how you feel about your sexuality, from celebratory to frustrated to helpless.

rewrite the script

Sexual "scripts" are the mental models we carry, made up of our beliefs about how sex should work. Your ideal sexual women in chapter 5 were examples of the scripts. They're what your monitor is measuring you against when she begins to feel frustrated—and if those scripts contradict each other, you can imagine how confused and helpless and frustrated your monitor must get sometimes!

The scripts aren't about what we intellectually believe is true. You can disagree, intellectually or politically, with a script and still find yourself behaving according to it and interpreting your experience in terms of it. It serves as a subconscious template for your little monitor to filter and organize your experience, a template written into your brain long before you could develop your own ideas about how sex works.

In the English-speaking world before 1700 CE, the cultural script was that women were more sexually voracious than men and had to be controlled or else they'd run wild. That began to change, and by 1800, the script had flipped, and women were expected to be largely asexual—at least, educated, middle-class women were expected to be asexual. Poor women were still viewed as sexually insatiable, with, ahem, "uncontrolled animal instincts."

The script has evolved further over the twentieth and twenty-first centuries. You may recognize these modern cultural scenario scripts:

- "Men's sexuality is simple and women's sexuality is complex."
- "Women don't have as strong a sex drive as men."

- "Orgasm is central to a positive sexual encounter."
- "Sex is more emotional for women than for men."

Your experience of sexuality may match these scripts, or it may not. But by now, you know that people vary—that is, they're different from each other, and also they change across time.

When the script doesn't seem to match your experience, the script is wrong, not you.

For this exercise, write the narrative of the kind of sex you have. Don't judge it or compare it with anything else, just describe it as it is. Try on the idea that your sexuality, as it is right now, is the "ideal."

You'll experience dissonance as you do this. That's okay—in fact, it's the goal. In particular, notice the places where you feel an urge to judge or criticize or feel bad about the sex you have. Highlight or underline them as you go, or reread the narrative when it's written and mark the places where you notice critical reactions in your thoughts or feelings.

Her (your) name is: _____

What does this ideal, real woman look like, and how does she behave outside sexual situations?

How does she initiate sex, if she does?

What does she do and how does she feel during sex?

How does her partner feel about her sexuality?

What would she *never* do or experience?

[blank box]

Did you spot aspects of your sexuality that violated your internal monitor's expectancy of how sex is supposed to work, or places where you felt self-critical, judgmental, or frustrated? Great! In the next exercise you'll practice noticing that kind of emotion and releasing it.

Your best source of knowledge about your sexuality is your own internal experience. When you notice disagreement between the script and your body's experience—and everyone does, at some point—always assume *your body is right*. And assume everyone's body is different from yours, as are everyone's scripts.

from the q & a vault

Q: **How do you get over performance anxiety?**

A: Performance anxiety happens when there is some standard, some aspirational ideal against which you're comparing yourself, or some expectation you believe your partner has that you're supposed to live up to. So to overcome performance anxiety, change your relationship with those standards and expectations.

The how-to is familiar by now: mindfulness practice. Turn your attention toward the pleasure happening in your body and/or your partner's, and when your attention slides into anxiousness, with those assessments of whether or not you're meeting some standard or expectation or some aspirational ideal, just notice those thoughts and feelings, say hello, and let them know you're busy right now paying attention to pleasure. Set them aside for the time being and return your attention to sensation. Repeat. Again. And again.

When you first try this, it will work for approximately two seconds, then you'll immediately revert to comparing yourself with that aspirational ideal. That's normal. Just keep practicing, and the two seconds will expand to five seconds, then thirty seconds, then five minutes, and then thirty minutes.

As usual, it will probably be easier to practice on your own at first, then add a partner. And there's no need to get frustrated or impatient—each time you notice the anxiety, you win! You noticed! You interrupted it, rather than letting it escalate. And you returned your attention where you wanted it. Congratulations!

mindfulness

To assess the source of your sexual frustration, dissatisfaction, or distress, it's helpful to observe that distress neutrally, without judgment, worry, or upset. Which is a learnable skill. The most effective way to learn it is through the practice of mindfulness.

Reluctant beginners often ask, "Why would I practice being aware of what's happening now, when I *hate* what's happening now? Why should I stop judging now?"

The answer is: turning away from what's happening now is actually a barrier standing between you and a different now. Judging your sexual distress could even be a primary *cause* of your sexual distress. Mindfulness, you'll remember, is the practice of *nonjudgmental, present-centered awareness*, neutrally noticing what's happening in the here and now—even if what you're aware of is unpleasant.

Chapter 4 introduced a two-minute mindfulness practice using the breath. Chapter 8 included a "sensation" exercise that extended the mindfulness practice in both time and intensity. Here's a practice that's even more advanced.

Choose a body part to stretch. You might try touching your toes, either standing or sitting. You might stretch your glutes, your calves, your triceps, or your humerus (lower arm) muscles. It's up to you. Stretch your muscle of choice to the point that it feels a little uncomfortable but not painful.

Now the hard part: hold that stretch for forty-five seconds. As you stretch, tune your attention to the stretch sensation.

Your mind will wander to something else, of course. That's

normal. Just notice that your mind wandered, then gently redirect your attention back to the stretching sensation you're creating.

The sensation might grow or fade. Part of your body might start to shake or throb. You might notice an urge to stop, to make the sensation go away. Be patient and compassionate with every response you notice in your body, your thoughts, and your feelings. Just notice all of it, without doing anything.

Then give yourself fifteen to thirty seconds to rest.

Start with five repetitions the first time. Increase the number of repetitions each time, still noticing the sensation and the ways your body and mind respond to it. In the research on stretch sensation and muscle extensibility, participants stretch this way for a full thirty minutes!

The most astonishing consequences of a simple (yet challenging) mindfulness exercise like this is how readily your brain transfers the skill of neutrally noticing an uncomfortable *physical* sensation to neutrally noticing an uncomfortable *emotional* sensation. A practice like this helps you learn to step outside of uncomfortable feelings and notice them neutrally, rather than panicking or ignoring them or denying them, all of which will simply intensify the discomfort in the long run. When you can turn with compassion and kindness toward whatever discomfort you're experiencing, you can begin to help your frustrated or helpless monitor solve problems more effectively.

For those struggling with sexual distress like painful sex, diminished desire or pleasure after a medical issue (such as gynecological cancers or a traumatic experience of childbirth), or mental health issues like depression and anxiety, delving deeper into mindfulness could be the most helpful approach to addressing these difficulties.

what happens in the magic circle

In chapter 7, we described the protected space created by couples who sustain strong sexual connections—a "magic circle" where they leave behind their daily lives and connect sexually with each other. In that chapter, the goal was to understand how we can transition from our everyday lives into that magic circle.

Here, we want to explore what can happen once we're in it.

Because what can happen is magical. And it defies any script anyone has ever written.

Magic circles are a psychosocial space where we experience two essentials of human life: ritual and play. Play is consequence-free practice for our adventures out in the world. Ritual reconnects us with home, including feelings of safety and comfort. Sex can be play, and it can be a ritual. We lay our bodies down together, skin to skin, and we find our way home. We rub our genitals together and touch our mouths to someone else's mouth or skin or genitals or feet, and we play.

In this exercise, you'll imagine sexual encounters as ritual and as play.

Sex as Ritual. Rituals are typically structured, repeating the same formal actions—sometimes even word for word, gesture for gesture—each time. They may celebrate specific occasions, like holidays, or they may be rites of communion practiced to reinforce people's sense of connection with something larger than themselves or simply a form of homecoming.

Describe a sexual experience that involves entering the magic circle–ritual style—following a structure to honor a special occasion or to reinforce a sense of connection. You may choose to use an example of ritual sex you've experienced in real life, or you may prefer to imagine a ritual you might enjoy, including what you might be honoring and how you might honor it.

In what contexts might you most value ritual-style (rather than play-style) sex? (Examples: scheduled sex that happens regularly; sex right before or right after a long separation; spontaneous sex; sex when you're tired or when you're feeling great; sex on vacation; sex early in a relationship or decades into a relationship.)

Sex as Play. Play comes in two main varieties: *rough-and-tumble play*, like sports or horseplay, and *story play*, like playing pretend or role-play. Both types involve improvisation and exploration, trying new things in the expectation that partners in play will assert their curiosity and sense of adventure, and they will communicate clearly if something pushes them outside the magic circle.

Describe a sexual experience that involves entering the magic circle play style. You may choose to use an example of playful sex you've experienced in real life, or you may prefer to imagine play you might enjoy, including the story or the rough-and-tumble you might engage in.

In what contexts might you most value play-style (rather than ritual-style) sex?

As always, you may choose to pursue these kinds of encounters or not. You may choose to share them with a partner or keep them to yourself. It's your imagination, your body, and your choice. Never forget: sex positivity means each person gets to choose how they feel about their body and how and when they share their body—and their thoughts and feelings—with anyone else.

two objects

The final exercise in this workbook is one I learned from sex thera-pist Gina Ogden. She asked her clients to bring to their sessions two objects. Here's how she explained it in her book, *Exploring Desire and Intimacy*:

> One object is to represent a part of your sexual story you want to keep, nurture, and expand. The other object is to represent a part of your sexual story that you want to release and move beyond.

With all that you know about your sexual past and your sexual present, choose an object that makes tangible the aspects of your sexuality you want to allow to grow, and choose another object that makes tangible the aspects of your sexuality you want to let go. Don't get bogged down in the choice; give yourself five minutes to consider and choose two. They don't have be The Perfect Object; they just have to represent something you want to keep and some-thing you want to release.

Now physically touch the first object, explore it with curiosity and compassion, notice how you feel. Connect with it as if it were an old and beloved friend.

Write down what the object represents, what made you choose it. Explain how this aspect of your sexuality came to be. What confluence of circumstances came together to create this part of you?

Then take a few minutes to write a letter to the object, thanking it for the good things it has brought your life, and your hopes and wishes for its future with you:

You can use the "creating change" worksheets from chapter 3 to make a plan for how you'll allow that.

Now touch the second object, explore it with the same curiosity and compassion you had for the first one. Notice how you feel. Connect with it from a slight distance, as if it were a former partner from long ago, with whom you shared some intense conflict, though you've released the pain and moved forward in your life.

Write down what the object represents, what made you choose it. Explain how this aspect of your sexuality came to be. What confluence of circumstances created this part of you?

Then take a few minutes to write a letter to the object, thanking it for the lessons it brought your life. Think of it as a farewell letter. This object has served you, helped you grow in ways that perhaps you didn't even know you could grow. Thank it for what it brought you, recognizing that this object did not choose to be a source of pain:

Again, if you like, you can use the "creating change" worksheets from chapter 3 to make a plan for how you'll allow that aspect of your sexuality to move out of your life.

one important thing

Take a moment to look back at the exercises in this chapter. Write down one important thing you learned, whether it's about sex in general or about your sexuality in particular:

conclusion

In my decades as a sex educator, I have found that the ideas in this workbook help people to imagine a sexuality for themselves that is outside the cultural script. For thirty years or more, science has been writing this new, evidence-based script that allows for all the ways we vary from one another and change across our life spans. When we embrace this new way of understanding ourselves and our partners, we open the door to maximal sexual wellbeing. This new script tells us:

- We're all made of the same parts, organized in different ways.
- There's a sexual accelerator *and a brake*.
- Pleasure, desire, and genital response are not the same thing.
- Arousal nonconcordance is normal.
- Responsive desire is normal.
- And, perhaps above all, *context* shapes our access to pleasure.

I encourage you to share the ideas, exercises, and lessons in this workbook with friends and family. Talk with your daughter or your mother about the different "ideal sexual women" that have been prescribed to you by your culture, across generations. Talk with your best friend about the wide variety of orgasms you've had—good and bad. Talk with your partner about the contexts that facilitate maximum pleasure and the strategies you can implement together, to create those contexts.

At the end of *Come As You Are*, I wrote about the animated movie *Kung Fu Panda*. It's about a cartoon panda named Po, who does kung fu. In the course of his training, he is offered "the dragon scroll," purported to hold the "key to limitless power," the secret ingredient for greatness.

To his disappointment, when he unrolls the scroll he discovers it is blank; it's just a mirror, reflecting his face.

Then he has his revelation: "There is no secret ingredient. It's just you."

Sexuality is about so much more than any single book can capture, but in the end great sex comes down to one fairly simple idea: the secret ingredient . . . is you.

The purpose of this workbook is to hold a mirror up to your sexuality and allow you to see it differently, to see the greatness that exists, so you can embrace it. There is no "secret ingredient" that makes great sex great—except you. The secret ingredient is *you*.

acknowledgments

S. Bear Bergman helped me write the section "No Two Alike for Trans, Intersex, and Nonbinary Folks" in chapter 1. Gratitude to him for helping make a workbook for women a little more welcoming for people outside the binary, who are just as deserving of great sex.

Gratitude to Petra Zebroff for her support in including the Sexual Initiation Scale of Arousal, which makes concrete and practical so many of the abstract concepts from *Come As You Are*. May it be shared far and wide!

Gratitude to the beta readers who provided crucial feedback: Amelia Pantalos, Aricka Harveland, Kat Stark, Kitty May, Liza Hanks, Shaun Miller, Stephanie Ellis, and Teal Dye, along with the attendees of my Esalen workshops and others who prefer to be anonymous. Thank you so much!

Gratitude to the brilliant and thoughtful Lindsay Edgecombe, my literary agent, who said, "What about a *CAYA* workbook?" You are the best.

Gratitude, too, to Julianna Haubner, the workbook's editor. Thank you for being gentle yet ruthless.

And gratitude to the hundreds of therapists, medical providers, educators, coaches, and other professionals who've shown me how they're using *Come As You Are* with their clients, patients, and students. Your ideas helped me create a tool that I hope will help you and your colleagues change people's lives for the better. I did not anticipate that *CAYA* would resonate with providers the way it has, and connecting with so many of you who share my vision of a world full of pleasure and free of pain and shame has been one of my greatest joys since *CAYA* was published.

recommended reading

part 1: the (not-so-basic) basics

one: anatomy: no two alike
Woman: An Intimate Geography, by Natalie Angier

two: the dual control model
Human Sexuality and Its Problems, by John Bancroft

three: context
Come As You Are, by Emily Nagoski

part 2: sex in context

four: emotional context
It's Not Always Depression: Working the Change Triangle to Listen to the Body, Discover Core Emotions, and Connect to Your Authentic Self, by Hilary Jacobs Hendel
Why Zebras Don't Get Ulcers, by Robert Sapolsky

five: cultural context
Things No One Will Tell Fat Girls, by Jes Baker
The Body Is Not an Apology, by Sonya Renee Taylor

part 3: sex in action

six: arousal
Come As You Are, by Emily Nagoski

seven: desire
Better Sex through Mindfulness, by Lori Brotto
How Sexual Desire Works, by Frederick Toates

part 4: ecstasy for everybody

eight: orgasm
Becoming Orgasmic, by Julia Heiman and Joseph LoPiccolo
Urban Tantra, by Barbara Carrellas

nine: a new script
Better Sex through Mindfulness, by Lori Brotto
Exploring Desire and Intimacy, by Gina Ogden

more topics

relationships
The Seven Principles for Making Marriage Work, by John Gottman
Hold Me Tight, by Sue Johnson
When Someone You Love Is Polyamorous, by Elisabeth Sheff

for people who are underrepresented in research and media

Big Big Love, by Hanne Blank

Black Women, Sex and the Lies our Mothers Told Us, by Hareder T. McDowell

Girl Sex 101, by Allison Moon

The Ultimate Guide to Sex and Disability, by Cory Silverberg, Fran Odette, and Miriam Kaufman

for young people

Sex Is a Funny Word, by Cory Silverberg

Drawn to Sex, by Erika Moen

S. E. X., by Heather Corrina

for different life stages

The Fourth Trimester, by Kimberly Ann Johnson

Like a Mother, by Angela Garbes

The Menopause Book, by Barbara Kantrowitz and Pat Wingert

The Wisdom of Menopause, by Christiane Northrup

better know the science

Health at Every Size, by Linda Bacon

The Psychophysiology of Sex, edited by Erick Janssen

The Science of Trust, by John Gottman

The Polyvagal Theory, by Stephen Porges

for professionals

The Principles of Pleasure: Working with the Good Stuff as Sex Therapists and Educators, by Laura Rademacher with Lindsey Hoskins

An Introduction to Sexuality Education: A Handbook for Mental Health Practitioners, by Karen Rayne and Ryan Dillon

Exploring Desire and Intimacy: A Workbook for Creative Clinicians, by Gina Ogden

about the author

Emily Nagoski, Ph.D., is the author of *Come As You Are: The Surprising New Science That Will Transform Your Sex Life* and co-author of *Burnout: The Secret to Unlocking the Stress Cycle*. She has been a sex educator for more than two decades.